I0055677

Uncertainty

Decision-Making and Team Work
in High-tech Healthcare

PERSON-*SoulMindBody*-HOOD
& Relational Medicine

Uncertainty

Decision-Making and Team Work in High-tech Healthcare

PERSON-*SoulMindBody*-HOOD & Relational Medicine

Federica Raia
Murray Kwon
Mario Deng

University of California, Los Angeles, USA

World Scientific

NEW JERSEY · LONDON · SINGAPORE · BEIJING · SHANGHAI · HONG KONG · TAIPEI · CHENNAI · TOKYO

Published by

World Scientific Publishing Co. Pte. Ltd.

5 Toh Tuck Link, Singapore 596224

USA office: 27 Warren Street, Suite 401-402, Hackensack, NJ 07601

UK office: 57 Shelton Street, Covent Garden, London WC2H 9HE

British Library Cataloguing-in-Publication Data
A catalogue record for this book is available from the British Library.

UNCERTAINTY, DECISION-MAKING AND TEAM WORK IN
HIGH-TECH HEALTHCARE
PERSON-*SoulMindBody*-HOOD & Relational Medicine

Copyright © 2023 by World Scientific Publishing Co. Pte. Ltd.

All rights reserved. This book, or parts thereof, may not be reproduced in any form or by any means, electronic or mechanical, including photocopying, recording or any information storage and retrieval system now known or to be invented, without written permission from the publisher.

For photocopying of material in this volume, please pay a copying fee through the Copyright Clearance Center, Inc., 222 Rosewood Drive, Danvers, MA 01923, USA. In this case permission to photocopy is not required from the publisher.

ISBN 978-981-125-467-3 (hardcover)
ISBN 978-981-125-468-0 (ebook for institutions)
ISBN 978-981-125-469-7 (ebook for individuals)

For any available supplementary material, please visit
https://www.worldscientific.com/worldscibooks/10.1142/12788#t=suppl

Typeset by Stallion Press
Email: enquiries@stallionpress.com

SHORT SUMMARY

Grounded in the insight that "High-tech medicine is forcing new territories for humans to dwell in," in 2015, we published our conceptual and methodological framework "Relational Medicine — Personalizing Modern Healthcare: The Practice of High-Tech Medicine as a Relational *Act*." We build on this framework and put it to work in "Uncertainty, Decision-Making and Team Work in High-tech Healthcare: PERSON-*SoulMindBody*-HOOD & Relational Medicine." This book presents a fully developed single case analysis consisting of recorded consecutive encounters in a dramatically accelerating life-and-death decision-making situation in the high-tech medical practice of Advanced Heart Failure (AdHF) in a teaching hospital.

We analyze the recorded medical encounter interactions during which practitioners, patient, and family face multiple uncertainties as a decision-making process unfolds, and the patient's condition changes. We show how an interprofessional team — AdHF cardiologist, AdHF surgeon, coronary care unit nurse, and Fellows — discuss AdHF life-prolonging options with their patient and family. We make visible the essential roles of each multidisciplinary team member in helping frame for the patient and family what it is that is going on and the changing available options while attending to the patient's soul-mind-body. In bringing different data, perspectives, and facets of understanding to bear, this book offers a novel approach to study high-tech medical care grounded in the actual everyday practice. Using a micro-ethnographic data analysis, we unravel a heretofore unrecognized universe of practice themes and present suggestions for medical education and training aimed at continuous reflections on practice improvement.

ACKNOWLEDGMENTS

Many people have contributed to the current book. The Raia Relational Ontology & Phenomenology of Practice lab team at UCLA worked for years tirelessly on this case analysis. Former and current team members include Naa'im Eggleton, Srikanth Krishnan, Jennifer Plotkin, Nadine Tanio, and Irina Silacheva.

Federica's Raia Care Learning and Becoming Lab (the C_LaB), a qualitative data analysis interest group composed of education researchers, linguist anthropologists, medical practitioners, and students provided additional space to discuss the methodological as well as practice-related issues relevant to this book. Special thanks go to the participants including Marjorie H Goodwin, Julia Katila, Srikanth Krishnan, Lezel Legados Irina Silacheva, Ana Elvira Steinbach Torres, Siraj Sodhi, and Menelik Tafari.

The numerous residents in Mario Deng's monthly lecture "Decision-Making in Advanced Heart Failure" and multidisciplinary nursing team members, specifically Moira Kelly, in the Ronald-Reagan UCLA Medical Center Critical Care Unit (CCU) were instrumental in critically advancing the research team's analytical and conceptual thought process.

The UCLA cross-campus cross-school project would not have been possible without the leadership support of the School of Education & Information Studies (EI&IS), David Geffen School of Medicine (DGSOM) and UCLA Health.

Inspiration continued to come from the Relational Medicine Foundation, namely Candace Moose, Jim Moose, and Victoria Groysberg; our patients and their families; Brent and Tracy Shubin; and our families, specifically our beloved mothers Liliana Monaco, Su Yong Kwon and Eva Deng.

For her continuous support and encouragement and her constructive and insightful comments, we thank Professor Marjory (Candy) H. Goodwin.

Federica's mentor and spiritus rector Professor Charles (Chuck) Goodwin was — before and after his untimely passing — a continuous inspirational interlocutor.

ABOUT THE AUTHORS

Federica Raia, PhD, is associate professor at UCLA in the School of Education and Information Studies (SE&IS) and in the David Geffen School of Medicine at UCLA (https://seis.ucla.edu/faculty-and-research/faculty-directory/federica-raia).

Her work focuses on studying professional practices of care in Medical and Education contexts where professionals, albeit in the specificity of each situation and community, confront the complex and important question of *How to care for the Other* in need to develop a new and meaningful sense of being in the world. Her work is situated at the crossroads of learning, sciences and technology, and the concept of personhood. It is informed by complexity science and continental philosophy, in particular, Martin Heidegger's and Maurice Merleau-Ponty's philosophical work on fundamental ontology and phenomenology of the lived experience always embedded in the world we inhabit, always in interaction with equipment, tools, and other persons.

She has developed a conceptual framework called *Relational Ontology*. Within this framework she focuses on the relational aspect of encountering the Other in asymmetrical power and knowledge distribution situations as it is the case in teacher/student and doctor/patient encounters. As discussed in her work, in the professional practices of both educators and healthcare practitioners, the ethical imperative to care is part of the social positioning (1) manifested in the world inhabited by the professionals in caring for the Other and (2) toward oneself, taking a stand on one's own path of becoming this kind of practitioner.

Dr Raia studies practices at the interactional level. The ethnographic microanalyses of audio-video recorded interactions make visible:

- What it means to care for the Other
- What it means to "notice" in practice

- What it means to be and become a practitioner in high-tech medicine multiactivity practice of teaching/learning and patient care
- The multimodality of learning and practicing as a process of becoming
- The background skills, the "know how" utilized in communication practices that create the possibility of comportment

Murray Kwon, MD, is associate clinical professor of Surgery and an American Board of Thoracic Surgery certified Thoracic and Cardiac Surgeon. After completing his undergraduate education at UC Berkeley (BA 1988), Medical School at Northwestern University Medical School (MD 1996) and a business degree at Kellogg Graduate School of Management (MBA 1996), Dr Kwon completed General Surgery Residency (1996–1998, 2001–2004), Cardiac Research Fellowship (1998–2001), and Cardiothoracic Surgery Residency (2004–2007) at Stanford University before joining UCLA for a Cardiothoracic Transplantation Fellowship (2007–2008). Subsequently, Dr Kwon was appointed as UCLA faculty, and is currently the Surgical Director of the UCLA Mechanical Circulatory Support Device Program.

Mario Deng, MD, professor of Medicine, is a cardiologist, specialized in the care of patients with advanced heart failure, mechanical circulatory support devices, and heart transplantation. After medical training in Germany and a postdoctoral cardiology research fellowship at Stanford University, he served as the Medical Director of the Interdisciplinary Heart Failure & Heart Transplantation Program at Muenster University (1992–2000), Director of Cardiac Transplantation Research at Columbia University (2000–2011), and Medical Director of the UCLA Integrated Advanced Heart Failure/Mechanical Support/Heart Transplant program (2011–2016) (http://www.uclahealth.org/MarioDeng).

As principal investigator/joint-principal investigator of continuously since >25 years federally, philanthropy- and industry-funded translational systems biology projects, Dr Deng codeveloped the first diagnostic leukocyte gene expression profiling test in transplantation medicine that gained United States Food and Drug Administration (USFDA)-regulatory clearance to rule out rejection without tissue biopsies (AlloMap™). Based on this success, Dr Deng's lab was invited by the National Institutes of

Health (NIH)/US-Critical Illness and Injury Trials Group (USCIITG) to develop a molecular immunology blood test to better predict survival outcomes in patients with various phenotypes of advanced heart failure (*My*LeukoMAP™) that gave rise to the molecular startup company LeukoLifeDx. During the COVID-19 pandemic, Dr Deng's lab was awarded an NIH/National Institute of Allergy and Infectious Diseases (NIAID) grant in 2021 to develop a multidimensional immunology blood test to better predict long-term outcomes of COVID-19.

Embedding systems biological outcome precision prediction tools into the clinical framework of a humanistically sound high-tech modern medicine practice is reflected in Dr Deng's research collaboration with Professor Federica Raia (UCLA SE&IS and DGSOM) in the "Relational Medicine™" project. Together with Professor Raia, he developed the Relational Medicine Theory with the core concept of the Relational *Act* to improve the understanding and practice of modern medicine. In the context of this work, Professor Deng is the cofounder and copresident, with Professor Raia, of the Relational Medicine Foundation, a nonprofit organization in support of the ongoing collaboration among different stakeholders: patients, caregivers, healthcare providers, education researchers, and artists/theater professionals to improve the understanding and practice of high-tech modern medicine (http://relationalmedicinefoundation.org/).

CONTENTS

CHAPTER 1
INTRODUCTION

On January 27, 2012, the American Heart Association issued a scientific statement on decision-making in Advanced Heart Failure (AdHF) (Allen *et al.*, 2012) endorsed by the Heart Failure Society of America, the American Association of Heart Failure Nurses, and the Society for Medical Decision Making.

> Advanced heart failure, with its high degree of prognostic uncertainty and complex trade-offs in the choice of medical care, demands a thoughtful approach to communication and decision making. These interactions are not 1-time events but occur as an evolving series of discussions over time, particularly as a patient's condition changes. Such interactions may be difficult and time-consuming, and they often require planning to create a supportive environment for effective communication. (Allen *et al.*, 2012, p. 1939)

During the last 50 years, the rapidly expanding treatment options increased patients' life span and, consequently, the disease's duration. In this high-tech medical practice, patients are offered therapeutic options that were unthinkable 50 years ago. For example, the intervention option of heart transplantation requires the patient to live with a heart from somebody else; the Ventricular Assist Device (VAD) implantation option requires patients to live with their heart attached to a machine VAD or entirely substituted by a machine, an artificial heart (Raia & Deng, 2015b, 2016b). These life-saving therapeutic options change patients' as well as their family caregivers' life (Bidwell *et al.*, 2017; Brouwers Corline *et al.*, 2011; Dew *et al.*, 2001; Evangelista *et al.*, 2003; Kirklin *et al.*, 2015; Kitko *et al.*, 2015; Kitko Lisa *et al.*, 2020; Lefaiver, 2006; Magasi Susan *et al.*, 2019; Marcuccilli *et al.*, 2014; Ross *et al.*, 2010; Voltolini *et al.*, 2020). The *experiences of learning to live* tethered to a machine that is partly inside and partly outside one's body, attached to batteries that need to be changed every 4–12 h or with somebody else's heart are novel to patients and their family caregivers (Kitko *et al.*, 2015; Kitko *et al.*, 2020; K.Kostick *et al.*, 2019).

A shared decision-making process supported by decision aids to accept to live long term (Destination Therapy) with a Left Ventricular Assist Device (LVAD) remains complicated and challenging and is relatively independent of the knowledge attained by patients (Allen *et al.*, 2018) or caregivers (McIlvennan *et al.*, 2018).

The decision-making process about AdHF therapeutic options emerges for the professionals at the tension of different factors (Vucicevic *et al.*, 2018): prognostic uncertainty of the disease, risk of the intervention, the complexity of the treatment options, and the balance of needing to follow the legal doctrines of informed consent safeguarding the patient and needing to maintain humanistic aspects in the patient–clinician communication (Kunneman *et al.*, 2019; Raia & Deng, 2015b). As existential bodily experiences, these are unknown to the AdHF interprofessional team caring for patients with AdHF (Caldwell *et al.*, 2007; Goodlin *et al.*, 2004; Klindtworth *et al.*, 2015; Raia & Deng, 2015b; Strang *et al.*, 2014; You *et al.*, 2017).

This book addresses these issues as they are encountered in the medical practice of AdHF. It follows the process of decision-making as it develops between a patient, his family, and the AdHF team in the Coronary Care Unit (CCU) over a series of medical encounters during which the patient's condition changes. We address shared decision-making as a complex process developing over time in the high-tech medical practice of AdHF in a large university teaching hospital in southern California. We show how the complexity of the phenomenon emerges from interrelated dynamics among the following:

- The act of making decisions (Whitney *et al.*, 2004) that are life-changing (Conway *et al.*, 2013; Haddow, 2005; Mauthner *et al.*, 2012; Mauthner *et al.*, 2015; Raia & Deng, 2015b; Shildrick, 2012, 2015).
- The varying conditions often requiring urgency or emergency decisions to be made by professionals and patients and their families (e.g., Crossland *et al.*, 2019; Eckman *et al.*, 2015; Engelhardt *et al.*, 2016; Grant *et al.*, 2020; Hargraves *et al.*, 2016; Hess *et al.*, 2015; Karnieli-Miller & Eisikovits, 2009; Mihalj *et al.*, 2020; Morris *et al.*, 2018).

- The interprofessional AdHF team structure whose members (e.g., cardiologist, nurse, surgeon) have different and complementary types of professional expertise shaping their perceptions and actions (C. Goodwin, 1994), needs, and stances (Raia, 2018).
- The varying levels of professional expertise shaping graduate medical learner/trainee perceptions and actions (Gonzalo *et al.*, 2014; Morris & Blaney, 2013; Paradis *et al.*, 2016; Peters & ten Cate, 2014; Raia, 2018; Raia & Smith, 2020; Shetty *et al.*, 2021).
- The interpersonal interactions of each team member with patient and family (Kunneman *et al.*, 2019).
- The engagement of team members in multiactivity spaces in which patient care and teaching/learning are taking place simultaneously (Raia, 2018; Raia & Smith, 2020).

We begin from the end.

Introducing the Case

We begin by noting how professionals present our case at the University Hospital Annual Heart Failure Symposium; and how the same case is taught and discussed with medical trainees in a monthly lecture for the Residents in the same University Hospital.

The annual heart failure symposium

A hundred healthcare professionals from southern California caring for patients with AdHF have gathered at the [University Hospital] Annual Heart Failure Symposium. The participants have the opportunity to discuss the latest evidence-based medicine study results, the current practice guidelines implemented at the University Hospital, and the multidisciplinary approaches of caring for patients, and learn from patients' perspectives. Physicians of different specialties (cardiologists, cardiac surgeons, infectiologists, and psychiatrists), nurses, pharmacologists, ventricular assist device coordinators, transplant coordinators, social workers, care coordinators, patients, and their families are attending. Participants also have the opportunity to develop and deepen the professional bonds with other practitioners who take complementary roles in caring for patients as AdHF and primary care physicians, e.g., referring internists/cardiologists and tertiary care center specialists. The afternoon session of the symposium is entitled Multidisciplinary Approaches to Patient Optimization; Dr. D, one of the AdHF cardiologists from the University Hospital and coauthor of this book, opens the session with a talk entitled *Patient Perspectives*. A few minutes into his talk, Dr. D describes Mr Spencer's case:

> I want now to dive right into a specific situation, into a very specific moment of a specific situation, and share the thought process. For this case, the patient agreed to participate in our RelationalMedicine encounter research project, directed by Professor Raia. It's a participatory action research project in which our medical practice is audio- or videotaped, and therefore we can go through it together and in much more detail later, also inviting the patients to participate.

The slide shows the details of the research project we discuss in Chapter 2. Then, Dr. D introduces the clinical case of Mr Spencer:

> Mr. Spencer is a 50 year old man with rheumatoid arthritis [...] who presents to [name removed] Hospital with diplopia, some neurological symptoms, and fever.

Dr. D's pointer circles each symptom and Mr. Spencer's medical history while talking: rheumatoid arthritis (RA), latent tuberculosis (TB), double vision (diplopia), the right eye, and lip droop (neurological symptoms), two cardiac arrests from which he needed to be resuscitated.

> Mr. Spencer has a cardiac arrest, and an Impella[1] is placed emergently — a concept that Dr. Cri and Dr. Naz just talked about [during the morning session]. After his second cardiac arrest, he is transferred to the [Name] hospital, has a heart muscle biopsy.
> It turns out he has a condition called Giant Cell Myocarditis, which is, among the inflammatory heart muscle conditions, probably the most malignant kind of myocarditis and leads to death in the median range of two to six months.

---

[1] A short-term catheter-based heart support pump.

We initiate immunosuppressive therapy, which is the recommended therapy. But he doesn't respond within a week or so. Therefore, we feel we need to replace the heart. We agree to place him on the heart transplantation waiting list and decide that he probably needs, for the waiting time, a mechanical support device — those that Dr. Car and Dr. Art have talked about this morning.

I (FR) appreciate the references Dr. D makes to the previous talks at the symposium; they offer an insight into how medical and scientific issues discussed in the morning fit together for one case study, offering a view of the AdHF management. For example, Dr. Car and Dr. Art discussed the VAD implantation as therapy to bridge a patient to transplantation when too unstable to survive the waiting period until a heart become available. In Mr Spencer's case, the instability was related to the fast progression of Giant Cell Myocarditis disease. As a researcher, I have followed the case, taking field notes, recording, and analyzing the recorded interactions with my coauthors as participant researchers. I remember an organizational and emotional roller-coaster, as Mr Spencer also defined this time, with all the changes and decisions the team and Mr Spencer and his family were confronted with within a few days. Indeed, as Dr. D describes, from an initial improvement and stabilization, Mr Spencer's heart function worsens despite immunosuppression therapy. The AdHF team recommends the evaluation for heart transplantation, and M. Spencer has to accept the idea of living with somebody else's heart. However, a few days later, the fast progression of the disease makes Mr Spencer too unstable to wait for transplantation with current medical therapy. The team recommends the implantation of a combination of VADs as a bridge to heart transplantation. Mr Spencer — who, as Dr. D describes, is a religious and spiritual person, wary of any possible aggressive clinical action serving the sole purpose of prolonging the physical being — needs to consent to another complex surgery in high-tech medicine. He consents. The surgery is scheduled for a day later.

However, Dr. D continues specifying that to conduct the surgery with the particular VAD that Mr Spencer has accepted requires a more complex organization that takes up to 24 h. Based on this added time and the reoccurrence of life-threatening arrhythmias making the heart race at 190 beats per minute rather than 60–100 beats per minute, the team needs to immediately discuss the possibility, if necessary, to insert a short-term mechanical device: a Venoarterial Extracorporeal Membrane Oxygenator (VA-ECMO). This is a much less invasive procedure than VAD implantation and heart transplantation, but an additional step to bridge Mr Spencer safely to the VAD surgery:

> We needed to immediately also decide, if necessary, to have a short-term bridge to [VAD implantation] with the VA-ECMO. During the bedside encounter on January 1, the patient declines this third step 'as one step too far' in the context of his Christian religious belief system. With this decision, he opposes his wife, brother, and parents — who are all at the bedside — imploring him to consent to this third procedure as well. While this bedside conversation is going on, the patient develops another episode of ventricular tachyarrhythmias.

Mr Spencer, as Dr. D indicates in his slides, had already suffered from cardiac arrest caused by a form of arrhythmias that can become lethal, requiring resuscitation. In Mr Spencer's case, it requires VA-ECMO mechanical device implantation, the one he has declined. However, the ECMO team that can resuscitate the patient and also insert an emergency VA-ECMO arrives at the scene:

> The ECMO team is being called to the scene where the situation is deteriorating into an emergency situation. The [ECMO] team's request for Mr. Spencer's consent to VA-ECMO becomes more pressing. However, Mr. Spencer cannot bring himself to make that decision for the VA-ECMO.
> Now comes the situation I want to dive into. I am the AdHF Attending that day. And the note is very straightforward; everything in yellow [Dr. D. projects his medical note and points to the upper part of slide reported in Fig. 1.1].
> In other words, it doesn't reflect the complexity of the situation but just a routine encounter. This is what goes through my mind. I find it important to document the patient's preferences.

> AdHF Note [Year] 0101 Dr. [D]
> I have seen the patient and discussed the plan of care with the fellow. I am in agreement with the assessment of treatment plan as stated in this document. Specifically patient and family
>
> 1. Agree to proceed with HVAD-BiVAD (patient declines PVAD-BiVAD or TAH)
> 2. Requests if debilitating stroke or other life-limiting condition not futile continuation of life sustaining treatment.

Figure 1.1: This text is the — very abstract and factual — summary of the AdHF-note that Dr. D places in Mr. Spencer's chart on January 1.

Dr. D pauses his case presentation and asks the following question to the audience:

If Mr. Spencer would code now, who would:

Choice 1 — let him die peacefully in concordance with his expressed preferences, and who would
Choice 2 — let him pass out and become unconscious from the v-tach/v-fib, then turn to his wife — his surrogate decision-maker — standing next to him at the bedside and follow her advice to put Mr. Spencer on VA-ECMO as a short-term bridge to [VAD] and heart transplantation?

Dr. D asks to vote for choice one and then choice two. More than 60% of the respondents vote for option one and then . . .

We leave the symposium at this moment to return to it at the end of the book and now move to a few months later in the CCU conference room where Dr. D is presenting the same case in his monthly lecture for the residents.

A monthly lecture for the residents

Dr. D is about to start his lecture for the residents on the monthly CCU rotation. They have their lunch on the go while continuing to work. His lecture, Decision-Making in Advanced Heart Failure, is designed to be interactive, participatory, thought-provoking, and empowering.

Dr. D loads his presentation on the room's computer screen with the sentence: "I have several patients who have been cared for and presented with certain situations that are challenging in the moment of decision-making, and there is no right or wrong way." He presents Mr Spencer's case and the decision-making scenario. Dr. D details many of the concepts in AdHF he did not have to during the symposium, mindful of the participants' levels of knowledge in the field since often third- and fourth-year medical students attend the lectures;

then:

> My question to you is: you are the Attending heart failure cardiologist in the room, the patient is coding, the code is refractory, that is patient doesn't come back. The patient is about to lose consciousness. What would you do at that moment? Let's go around.

The first resident to respond reckons that if the team had time to discuss the VA-ECMO procedure and if the patient was lucid and had the capacity to fully understand the implications of that, then *"I think I HOPE that I would respect that and not put it in."* As I am, Dr. D is struck by the Resident's sentence that, in my notes, I marked, as I do here, in capital letters. Indeed Dr. D remarks, "you *hope* for yourself that you would," the Resident assents, "well said, it's good to hear the practitioner's uncertainty, and the ethical and emotional dilemma the team members often face."

The residents' responses all address the dichotomous decision-making branching point. If the patient is mentally competent to decide, then the physician must follow the patient's wishes. If the patient is not deemed competent, then the physician can invoke the surrogate decision-maker (i.e., Mr Spencer's wife) or, in the absence of a surrogate, it resorts to "the two Attendings" consent — two Attending physicians involved in the case consensually make a decision. A very difficult decision to make. Building on each other, the residents problematized the situation unveiling the emerging uncertainties they would need to consider and contend with in practice. They ask questions to recreate the discursive context within which the VA-ECMO possibility was discussed in the encounter.

> I think he was very clear, obviously thought of end-of-life before. Yeah, it sounds like he's a religious man, is without hesitancy, doesn't appear depressed or anything like that, and he doesn't want

it. Even though the wife is the proxy, should he not have decision-making capacity, a split second when he did have decision-making capacity, he was very explicit that he does not want it. So, you could argue to what extent he understands the risk of the procedure itself and the likely outcome, but you don't have time to discuss. But I think it would be I would feel not right with myself if I went for it.

He clearly didn't know, didn't understand the risks and benefits. Everything is so fast in emergencies, like, how could you not. He is going for a heart transplant?? How could you not? So that's what's weighing on the back of my mind, everything feels so fast. I don't know. I think I think I guess I would withhold, but I think if there was any inkling. So I'm trying to see how I could split this. But I guess I would withhold, but that would probably be a decision that would affect me for a long time.

Echo all that was said, especially like hoping they be able to make that decision because it's hard with everyone and the family in the room telling you to do something and you're saying not to.

I agree with a lot of the sentiments about not doing it based on his decision we talked about. I do think we're considering the capacity, some understanding. We always say that there are some benefits that the patient understands. And I think for something as complicated as this, there's no possible way that someone who is not a medical professional would understand all of the intricacies of this sort of therapy. And, I think it's beneficial that you and the other people were there at the bedside because we want to keep in context the conversations that have been had to that point in terms of not just whether to say yes or no to the questions but what the intentions of his answers were. And so, it sounded like intentions were not wanting other devices, with not wanting to be walking with things outside his body and being ok with them on the inside.

Is there another option?

Organization of the book

Chapter 2 discusses the conceptual framework — research methodology and theoretical underpinning, guiding our ethnographic and participatory research work. We describe the iterative research model we have developed to study *practice* (Raia & Deng, 2015b), the microethnographic approach to studying the taped interactions. We take a critical discourse analysis approach to the persons-in-interaction *within* the social–institutional context because there is an uneven and dynamic distribution of power, needs, and knowledge. We introduce two aspects, *framing for* and *with the Other* and *uncertainty* in the medical decision-making process, necessary to make sense of the development of the clinical interactions. The goal is to allow the reader to follow the conversation and show how the decision-making process develops over time as a *collaborative effort among stakeholders* and analyze the complex interaction pattern in intra/interprofessional communication (with different healthcare practitioners) and interpersonal communications (with patient and family).

To make sense of what happened on January 1, we go back to see how the relationships and communication patterns between Mr Spencer, his family, and the AdHF team develop. We start from those days when Mr Spencer was hospitalized in the CCU. In Chapters 3 and 4, we follow Mr Spencer and the AdHF team from December 24 until December 29 through Mr Spencer's diary excerpts, participants' reflections, and recorded data from the moment-to-moment interactions with the medical team in the CCU. The dialogue between Mr Spencer and the team unfolds in an uncertain and continually developing clinical situation during these days. Specifically, we show how organizing in a meaningful context different scenarios, possibilities, experiences, and course of the disease in AdHF for a patient (*framing*) makes visible how *uncertainty* emerges and is negotiated in the moment-to-moment interactions as an integral part of the practice.

Chapter 5 reports the microethnography of the encounter with a transition from an elective discussion, with a systematic discussion of options as seen in Chapters 3 and 4, to an urgent situation. We show how, when discussing options, the question–answer sequences differs from what has been reported in other institutional context of general medical practice. Specifically, we show that to make sense of the question–answer sequences, a Relational Ontology and Phenomenology of Practice (Raia, 2018) approach is required because the social/institutional identities are expressed not only by the epistemic claims enacted in turns of talk (Heritage, 2010). They are formed from the existential demand of being this person (Duranti, 2005; Throop, 2003) always relationally intertwined with the Other who is beyond our grasp (Lévinas, 1969; Raia & Deng, 2015b;

Throop & Zahavi, 2020), toward whom there is always responsibility (Lévinas & Nemo, 1985), and being *this* person caring for the Other (Raia, 2018, 2020).

In Chapters 6 and 7, the nature of decision-making changes from urgency into an emergency and is complicated by the necessity to rapidly decide to be prepared for the implantation of a life-sustaining short-term mechanical device. We arrive at the situation described at the symposium and in the Resident lecture and analyze the encounter in which a decision to accept the short-term bridge to a long-term bridge to transplantation is imminent. How can Mr Spencer's *sense of personhood — integrating soul, mind, and body —* be safeguarded to make this life/death decision? How do the bodies of expertise distinguishing each participant's perceptions and actions (Goodwin, 1994) shape both teamwork, intra/interprofessional, and interpersonal communication? How are the tensions navigated and resolved during teamwork?

In Chapter 8, we summarize our work and discuss its implication for teamwork and Graduate Medical Education Programs (Residency and Fellowship) in the specific practice domain of AdHF with its Heart Failure and Transplantation Fellowship Program from the perspective of the practitioners as participant researchers.

CHAPTER 2
CONCEPTUAL FRAMEWORK

The heart, since ages, has occupied a place in people's imagination, poetry, songs, and everyday talk (Webb 2010). A secret, unique site where love is produced, where the soul originates and performs its operation. A non-localizable nonreplaceable site from which also language can specify and intensify attitudes, moods, feelings, and dispositions (Ochs & Schieffelin, 2009).

The heart, after the first heart transplantation, performed on December 3, 1967, in Kapstadt by Dr. Christiaan Barnard, the first implantation of a left ventricular assist device (LVAD) in 1984 and wearable mechanical circulatory support (MCS) devices (e.g., a total artificial heart completely substituting a person's heart) in 1994, has taken another form in the imagination of humanity: science, technology, and medicine had reached a stage where a diseased organ could be replaced by another biological one (Fig. 2.1a), or by a machine (Fig. 2.1b): a diseased organ, a localizable and replaceable heart.

The replaceable heart, as the gift of life (Healy, 2006) to give willingly and receive as an inherently nonreciprocal gift (Fox & Swazey, 1974a), always maintains a long-lasting connecting thread between those who pursue the exchange (Mauss, 2000). This heart opens possibilities of discourses, dichotomous, contradictory, and with sharply defined categories of embodiment: the competing needs, on the one hand, to personalize and, on the other hand, to objectify organs and bodies (Sharp, 1995) revealing the grafted organ and or the machine as an intrusion into, an addition to, or a replacement of, the body and the self (Fox & Swazey, 1974b; Haddow, 2005; Lock, 2002; O. F. Mauthner et al., 2015b; Raia, 2020; Raia & Deng, 2015b; Ross et al., 2010; Sharp, 1995, 1996, 2006; Shildrick et al., 2009; Shildrick, 2011, 2015) deeming high-tech medicine as a practice of spare-parts surgery (Shildrick et al., 2009).

Oh, gift-of-life-localizable-replaceable-transportable heart, in the body made of disposable commodities, are you opening us to the world of

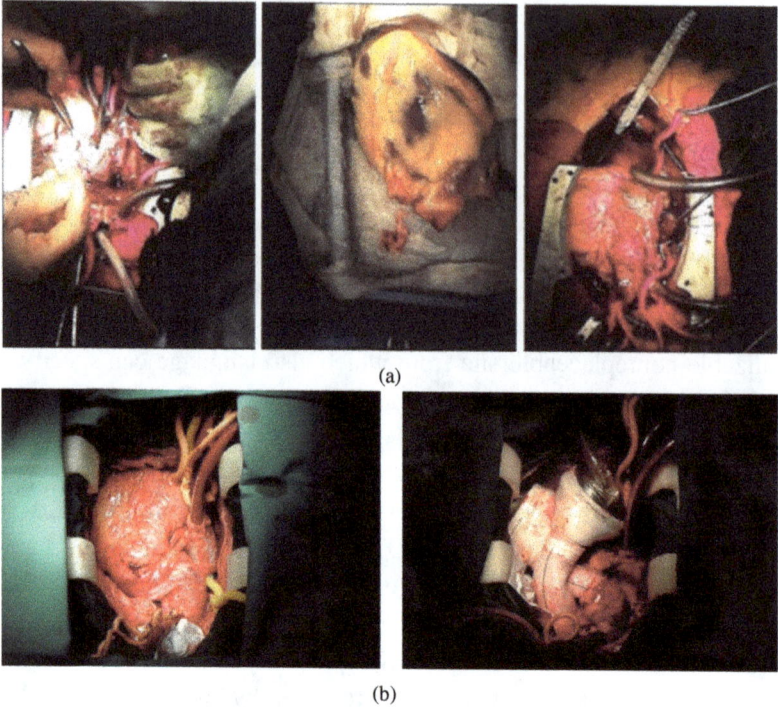

Figure 2.1: Replacing the heart. (a) Photo taken by heart surgeon. Dr. S, during heart transplantation upon a patient's request to document the placement of his "the new heart." The donor heart (center) replaces the patient's own heart (modified from Raia & Deng, 2015b). (b) Replacement of the patient's own heart (left) with a mechanical one, the Total Artificial Heart (Syncardia Systems Inc., Tucson, AZ) (right). View from the patient's head in the operating room. Modified from Raia and Deng (2015b).

technicity that according to Heidegger is overpowering and uprooting us from this earth and moving us closer to immortality? Martin Heidegger, in an interview with Der Spiegel responds to the question of why we should be concerned by technicity[1]:

> Everything functions. That is exactly what is uncanny [unheimlich]. Everything functions, and the functioning drives us more and more

---

[1]Martin Heidegger, in the interview for Der Spiegel in 1966 published posthumously in 1977. By technicity, Heidegger intends a way of being that discloses to us other beings only as quantifiable, disposable, and accumulable. Translation is modified from William J. Richardson SJ: http://www.ditext.com/heidegger/interview.html.

toward further functioning, and technicity dislodges people and uproots them from the earth [. . .]. All our relationships have become merely technical ones. It is no longer on earth that human beings dwell today [. . .] The poet [René Char], who certainly cannot be suspected of sentimentality or a glorification of the idyllic, said to me that the uprooting of human beings which is going on now is the end if thinking and poetizing do not acquire nonviolent power once again.

Undoubtedly, the gift-of-life-localizable-replaceable-transportable-functional-heart is opening new territories for humans to dwell in, but how do they show up as a phenomenon to recognize and study? To be entirely eradicated in the dreadful time of technicity (Heidegger, 1976), we must be solicited by those events and things that embody and further our understanding of being in the *technicity* paradigm: everything must make sense in terms of functionality and efficiency and things are understood and valued for their ability to be extracted, stockpiled, transported, and consumed. Are we? Sociology, political science, and critical education scholars have been pointing to the impact of politically legitimized neoliberal economic globalization on science (Moore *et al.*, 2011) and the reorganization of both health systems (Numerato *et al.*, 2012) and universities (See Bok, 2009; Torres, 2008). Threatened in their financial survival within technologically complex, knowledge-based economies, higher education institutions and hospitals have to adhere to managerial requirements of efficiency, functionality, profitability, and productivity. In medicine, these affect the healing relationship between health professionals and patients (Blanch, 2014; Gishen, 2020; Pellegrino, 1999). However, pockets of resistance (Butler, 1997; Foucault, 1990) express a different understanding of what it means to practice and to be a practitioner. In the shared spaces of high-tech Advanced Heart Failure (AdHF) practice, the technological project (see also Nicolini, 2006, 2010 for telemedicine innovation) that is challenging things and spaces to ultimately show themselves ready, definable, and accountable is disrupted.

Breakdown of Familiarity

The experiences of a person in interaction with scientific and technological advances such as living with an artificial heart or a heart from another person are novel and disruptive. Indeed, ethnographic and phenomenological studies (Sharp, 2006; Shildrick *et al.*, 2009) show that patients' and families' biographical accounts are punctuated by life events before and after the machine implantation/heart transplantation marking these events as interruption, as breakdown of a sense of a historic self, rooted in an existential past and projected in future possibilities of being the same person, the existential–temporal–horizon (Raia, 2020). Patient and family find themselves catapulted into a new world that is unfamiliar.

In previous work (Raia & Deng, 2015b), we studied medical interactions in the Cardio-Thoracic Intensive Care Unit (CTICU) between physicians and patients who are recovering from heart transplantation or from a mechanical Biventricular Assist Device (BiVAD) surgery and compared the disorientation and fear experienced by patients as similar to that of Dante, in the *Divine Comedy*, when he found himself lost in the *selva oscura* (dark forest). We demonstrated that it is the uncovering of the functional aspects of one's body — or of the loved one's body — and organs that makes it possible to accept the idea of a substitution of a permanently broken heart by heart transplantation or a substitution of part of the heart's pumping function by LVAD/BiVAD implantation. The technological project mediates the person's life experience. It modifies the bodily perception of being in the world (Merleau-Ponty, 1962) by opening new hybrid spaces of existence located both inside and outside of one's body. As it is in the case of Mr Spencer, this can happen without warning, unpredictably, thrusting a person into an unknown, unfamiliar world. However, there is no reassembly of the person with the new parts, machines, organs; it is not a motor exchange process, but rather a reminder of inherent vulnerability of the participants — patient and family (Shildrick, 2012) and healthcare professionals (Raia & Deng 2015b).

Caring for the Other

Although issues of objectivity and objectification emerge in understanding, studying, and controlling things and other beings (Daston & Galison, 2009; Haraway, 1988; Harding, 2015), ethnographic work on caring for AdHF patients (Fox & Swazey, 1974b; Haddow, 2005; Lock, 2002; O. E. Mauthner *et al.*, 2015b; Raia, 2020; Raia & Deng, 2015b; Ross *et al.*, 2010; Sharp, 1995, 1996, 2006; Shildrick *et al.*, 2009; Shildrick, 2011, 2015) points to the ideological contradictions and the struggle it takes to care for patients who are living these experiences that are at the same time experiences of a broken part and of a threat to a person's existence. Medical practitioners in AdHF develop an understanding of patients' experiences as part of AdHF professional knowledge (Raia, 2018; Raia & Deng, 2015b; Sharp, 2006). Like family members exploring new ways of encountering the world (M. H. Goodwin & Cekaite, 2018; M. Goodwin, 2006; Goodwin Marjorie & Cekaite, 2013), in the practice of high-tech medicine of AdHF participants are mutual apprentices creating a public and common world of all collective existence. They *learn* from and with each other to make sense of it and how it is inhabited by the Other. They *learn to care* for the Other and for themselves.

Indeed, a caveat in Dante's journey in the dark forest is that his guide, Virgilio, has never walked through the *selva oscura* and needs to unfold a path together with Dante. The path (Raia, 2020) is built in iterations showing its dialogic character (Bakhtin, 1981). The physician points toward *possibilities* for the patient to develop *his or her* sense of the landscape where *his or her* path is unfolding, introducing a sequence of specific eventful events, including those life events of machine implantation/heart transplantation, as cornerstones upon which the patient can start orienting within the new existential–temporal–horizon.

In this book, through the analysis of recordings of sequences of medical encounters between Mr Spencer, his family and the AdHF team, we show how unprecedented actions emerge not as a cultural form in the epoch of *technicity* describing the world as functional things — valued for their ability to be extracted, stockpiled, transported, and consumed — but as ruptures of it. Like internal noise these ruptures are capable of inducing emergent patterns (Attali, 1985), ways-of-being that open possibilities for "*thinking and poetizing*" both necessary to help *framing with and for the Other* what it is that is going on and to capture what cannot be fully described and utterly specified.

Framing

As discussed in Deborah Tannen's edited book, *Framing in Discourse* (1993), the concepts of framing and frames in discourse can be traced back to two main traditions: an interactional tradition, in which communication is understood as a relational process that develops in face-to-face practices (Bateson, 1956/1972), and a cognitive tradition that sees frames as mental models and regards people as information processors (Minsky 1975).

In its original formulation by the anthropologist Gregory Bateson, a frame is the participants' sense of the nature of the activity in which they are engaged. He utilizes two analogies to explain the frame concept in communication: Venn diagrams and picture frames. Frame, as a Venn diagram, has a double function: to include elements within its borders and exclude those outside it. It organizes people's perception (framing), facilitating the understanding that what is "inside" is connected somehow. Similarly, like a picture frame, it organizes people's perception, orienting them not only to attend to what is within the frame but indicating that different ways are required to make sense of what is inside and outside the frame. "Framing" defines context that organizes perceptions of behavior, and shapes how something makes sense to participants (Bateson, 1956/1972). As a meta-communicative use of language, Erving Goffman later describes framing as a sense of "what is it that's going on here?" (Goffman, 1974), allowing contextualization, that is, the context within which events unfold and actions occur (C. Goodwin & Duranti, 1992).

For example, in chronic heart failure nursing telemedicine practices studies, Nicolini (2012) points to artifacts such as the therapy sheet framing the nurse sense-making. It organizes the patient's condition development in time and provides an overview of all the patient's critical parameters within which new test results can be understood and within which the discursive practice of the telemedicine call can develop.

In the pediatric medical encounter, Tannen and Wallat (1987) show linguistic evidence of different frames, in which activities such as the physical examination which they call "examination frame" or the pediatrician answering the mother's questions about the child's condition, which they call "consultation frame" organize discourse. They show that the pediatrician balances several competing and often conflicting linguistic frames. For example, when the mother of the child asks questions about the child's condition during the physical examination, the pediatrician needs to interrupt the "examination frame" in which the doctor was talking playfully with the child and answer the mother's questions in a "consultation frame" linguistic style, which excludes the child from the discourse.

The second tradition, developed within cognitive psychology and artificial intelligence (Minsky 1975), considers frames as cognitive structures that organize and interpret the external world by fitting perception and information into pre-learned schemas about reality. This understanding of frames as mental models and people as information processors is often used in medical education. In their work, examining linguistic evidence for the existence of frames in pediatric interactions described earlier, Tannen and Wallat (1987) also identify this second understanding of frame and refer to it as "knowledge schema." They show that different knowledge schemas of health and cerebral palsy between the pediatrician and the mother of a pediatric patient account for the mother's discomfort and her numerous questions that trigger the change in the activity we described earlier, from the physical examination of a pediatric patient into a consultation with the mother.

In our previous work (Raia & Deng, 2015b), we showed how expectations or knowledge schemas of health shape the medical encounter between doctor and patient. In the framework of the Relational*Act*, for a clinician, a high-quality (Raia & Deng, 2015b) encounter extends outside the temporal and spatial boundaries of a patient room. It starts with the *preparation phase*,[2] outside and before entering the patient room, by reviewing the most up-to-date clinical information and anticipating to meet *this* person, anticipating the mood, and visualizing the encounter with *this* person. This *preparation phase* creates a framework for comparison based on the most up-to-date clinical information, enabling the doctor to pick up on any discrepancy (or concordance) in the observed (experienced) situation of the encounter and to reliably and rapidly compare the expected and observed impressions. The expected/observed (anticipated/experienced) comparison can pertain to Evidence-Based Medicine (EBM) perspectives on how the patient is medically doing. It can also relate to caring for a person catapulted into a new and unfamiliar world and in need of developing a new sense of self in the world (Raia, 2020). For example, Raia and Deng (2015b) describe the contrasting relation anticipated/experienced in the case of an

---

[2]With a mixed-method study of primary care practices that promote clinicians' presence and focused attention to the encounter with patients, Zulman *et al.* (2020) confirm some of the same practices we described in high-tech medicine (Raia & Deng, 2015b), including the preparation phase.

AdHF Attending expecting a patient to be in an upbeat mood, feeling "victorious over death" (p. 79) having survived various episodes of lethal arrhythmias and open heart surgery with an excellent course of recovery postoperatively, but encountering a contrasting reality, which allowed the Attending to address the issue immediately.

Framing as Care for the Other

Raia (2018), building on Heidegger's fundamental ontology, demonstrates that framing in discourse develops within existential spaces in which practice-linked identities manifest in the specificity of the activity at hand. She investigates the phenomenon of participation in simultaneous activities of teaching and learning and patient care during collaborative teamwork practice within AdHF. She demonstrates how the passage from one activity to another changes the meaning of "what is it that is going on here" and positions participants differently with respect to one another, e.g., teacher/learner, doctor/patient, which changes the participants' accountability. Raia frames the context of "caring-for the-Other" at the interactional level in asymmetrical power and knowledge distribution situations. She shows the phenomenon of negotiating through these spaces to support the Other in developing a new practice-linked identity in AdHF (e.g., becoming an AdHF cardiologist, a heart transplant patient) while developing a meaningful sense of life in becoming this person.

In AdHF, patients and their families are confronted by at least three complex transformative situations requiring help in making sense of them. They need to make sense of existential experiences new to them; they need to learn about the disease and its management; they need to engage in decision-making processes when confronted by diverse therapeutic options. Medical professionals caring for them have to attend to their need both in their medical encounter and teaching in practices. They have to attend to the interactions of the persons they care for with other professionals, for example, in training novices of the practice (Raia, 2018).

We combine three complementary approaches and modes of understanding of framing to study the medical interactions, in which there is a need to care for the Other.

The first, called by Bateson "psychological framing" in his study of psychotherapy (1956/1972), points to the relationship between the way in which the patient handles a situation and the way in which the therapist manipulates its framing toward therapeutic ends. Identifying this relationship in the moment-to-moment interactions of the medical encounters can unveil how healthcare professionals utilize their power and authority to frame these experiences and care for patients and families catapulted in new and unknown ways of life.

In a second more recent formulation in the learning sciences (Richards *et al.*, 2020; Russ & Luna, 2013), framing is understood as the response to student thinking, as an attunement to, respect for, and engagement with the intellectual resources students bring to bear in disciplinary contexts. Within this formulation, the focus is on teachers' framing and how it affects the way in which teachers notice, interpret, and respond to students' scientific thinking (e.g., Richards *et al.*, 2020; Robertson, *et al.*, 2015). This understanding of framing, therefore, unveils the teachers' epistemological stance. It can be applied to teaching and learning situations in teaching hospitals where interns', residents', and fellows' learning is shaped by their medical and clinical teachers' framing. We translate this formulation into making sense of how healthcare professionals' framing affects their interactions with patients and family, making sense of disease and therapeutic options requiring learning different medical concepts and a different language specific to the medical disciplinary context.

The importance of framing is also discussed in the context of medical decision-making literature. In their analysis of decision-making models, Wirtz *et al.* (2006) point to the limitations of these models and identify the neglect to consider how therapeutic options are contextualized, framed by the physician, as one of the most substantial limitations. They reason that this limitation impedes the development of doctor–patient decision-making models and the understanding of decision-making practices.

In combining these three different approaches to framing our interest is to study and make visible how healthcare professionals care for patients and their family supporting them in making sense of "what is it that's going on here," learning to live a new life, owning novel experiences, and engaging in active participation in decision-making. We make visible "framing for the Other." Our approach is specifically important because in AdHF the process of decision-making "occurs as an evolving series of discussions over time, particularly as a patient's condition changes" (Allen *et al.*, 2012, p. 1939). Patients and families need to learn about the development of the disease, the changing therapeutic options, and their likelihood of being the best options for the given situation. All these together require the healthcare team members and patient and family to negotiate multiple sources of uncertainty.

Facing Uncertainty

Sir William Osler, Chair of the Department of Medicine at Johns Hopkins University, who developed the concept of residency and was the first to implement bedside training, states: "medicine is a science of uncertainty and an art of probability." It is with this quote that Dr. Caroline Wellbery (2010) opens her essay in the *Lancet* on the value of uncertainty having liberating rather than constraining effect of practicing within uncertainty. She points out that practicing within uncertainty creates spaces in which doctors and patients together can manage risk and in which doctors can support patients to cope with uncertainty about health and disease. Indeed, as eloquently put by the Communication scholar James Bradac (2001), "humans should recognize that the possibility of certainty or complete predictability is an illusion and that believing in this possibility is a product of an erroneous Western attempt to control nature" (p. 456).

The medical sociologist René Fox, in her seminal ethnographic study of medical school training and in-training physicians' struggle with uncertainty (Fox, 1957), showed that physicians in training deploy various strategies to cope with their emotional reactions to multiple sources of uncertainty — varying from lack of scientific data to ambiguity in applying that data to a particular case. Fox, describing herself as "a watcher, chronicler, and analyst of uncertainty in numerous medical settings," later reflects on her work: "The importance of uncertainty in modern medical practice as a theoretical concept, an empirical phenomenon, and a human experience was first impressed on me by my teacher, Talcott Parsons (Parsons, 1951, 2013). He also conveyed to me the paradox and poignancy — for both physician and patient — of the fact that our great twentieth-century progress in medical science and technology has helped to reveal how ignorant, bewildered, and mistaken we still are in many ways about health and illness, life and death" (Fox, 1980, p. 2).

Over the last 40 years, as Han and colleagues (2019) show, the volume of research and specifically the citation of uncertainty in the medical literature is growing exponentially. However, Simpkin and Schwartzstein (2016), reflecting on the culture of medicine, report that there is still "a deep-rooted unwillingness to acknowledge and embrace it. Embodied in our teaching, our case-based learning curricula, and our research is the notion that we must unify a constellation of signs, symptoms, and test results into a solution. . . . Too often, we focus on transforming a patient's gray-scale narrative into a black-and-white diagnosis that can be neatly categorized and labeled. The unintended consequence — an obsession with finding the right answer, at the risk of oversimplifying the richly iterative and evolutionary nature of clinical reasoning — is the very antithesis of humanistic, individualized patient-centered care. We believe that a shift toward the acknowledgment and acceptance of uncertainty is essential — for us as physicians, for our patients, and for our health care system as a whole. Only if such a revolution occurs will we thrive in the coming medical era" (p. 1713). The larger medical community has shared Simpkin's and Schwartzstein's sentiments. West and West (2002), in their editorial on the necessity to accept uncertainty in medical decision-making, share the concern that ignoring uncertainty is equivalent to "removing from the medical profession some important 'tools of the trade' and placing obstacles in their way" (p. 320). How and to which extent physicians tolerate uncertainty has been receiving growing attention in research during the last decades (e.g., Allman, 1985; Geller *et al.*, 1993; Han *et al.*, 2021; Hillen *et al.*, 2017; Kuhn *et al.*, 2009). Concerns have been raised about the greater tolerance of uncertainty required in the era of precision medicine, when physicians need to interpret and translate probabilities based on large-scale studies into medical treatment tailored to the individual characteristics of each patient (Hunter, 2016).

In their systematic review of tolerance of uncertainty in health and healthcare-related outcomes, Strout and colleagues (2018), while finding that there is substantial heterogeneity in methodological quality and approaches, show some consistent trends pointing to a significant correlation between uncertainty tolerance and physicians, patients' behavior and emotional well-being. Similar conclusions are reached for healthcare providers in training with and increasing number of studies and efforts in curriculum design and training in support of a higher tolerance for uncertainty in young generations of physicians (Bochatay & Bajwa, 2020; Cooke & Lemay, 2017; Farnan *et al.*, 2008; Geller *et al.*, 1990;

Han *et al.*, 2015a, 2015b; Ilgen *et al.*, 2019; Knight & Mattick, 2006; Luther & Crandall, 2011; Nevalainen *et al.*, 2010; Tonelli & Upshur, 2019; Wray & Loo, 2015; Zikmund-Fisher, 2013). Indeed, issues of tolerance of uncertainty seem to have a far-reaching impact. Wayne and colleagues (2011) surveyed seven consecutive medical school classes from 1999 to 2005, assessing attitudes toward underserved populations at matriculation and graduation. They found that medical students who were tolerant of ambiguity were significantly less likely to have declining attitudes toward the underserved. Indeed, treating populations with less financial resources and less access to healthcare creates a more complex, often novel, and uncertain course of action. More recent studies suggest that openness to diversity is significantly and positively associated with tolerance of ambiguity over time. A more recent study (Geller *et al.*, 2021) suggests that openness to diversity before medical school could foster the development of tolerance of ambiguity, inviting future research to explore whether changes in students' interest in working in an underserved community are related to the initial trainee openness to diversity.

From the earlier discussion, we can appreciate uncertainty as multi-faceted and emerging from different aspects of entering and being in the world of healthcare. In patient–doctor interactions, Braddock *et al.* (1997, 1999) analyze audiotaped patient–physician consultations to study decision-making in clinical interactions. They identify the discussion of uncertainties as one of the most critical elements for decision-making, crucial for a patient's understanding of the options and conceivably promoting trust and encouraging adherence to therapeutic management. Echoed by subsequent studies by McNutt (2004) and Kasper and colleagues (2008), they argue that informing patients about uncertainty in clinical and scientific evidence needs to be understood within an ethical dimension, and negotiation of uncertainties should not result in their reduction. Parascandola *et al.* (2002) show that medical uncertainty is so challenging to communicate that many physicians avoid disclosing and discussing or oversimplifying it. When physicians communicate uncertainty for risk and benefit of treatment, they limit the discussion about uncertainty to probabilities (Politi *et al.*, 2007) instead of offering patients necessary professional guidance to support patients and families in the complex decision-making process as suggested by West and West (2002).

In research concerned with the experience of illness, Kasper and colleagues (2008) utilize in-depth interviews of patients with cancer to explore the uncertainties associated with medical decisions that the patients face. They identify multiple sources of uncertainty pertaining to diagnoses, prognoses, and treatment of disease; patient's preferred degree of involvement, issues of patient social integration, and mastering of life requirements; and physician's competence and trustworthiness — which includes how risk information is provided and how the patient deciphers it. They argue that the range of uncertainties represented by these sources transcends the aspects of decision-making and conclude that these sources make uncertainty inherently constitutive of the patient–clinician interactions. In nursing research, Merle Mishel (1988) theorizes that persons construct meaning for illness events, with uncertainty as a cognitive state indicating the inability to determine the meaning of illness-related events. Importantly, rather than seeing uncertainty as something to be avoided and minimized, similarly to West and West (2002) and Simpkin's and Schwartzstein (2016), Mishel argues that uncertainty should be approached as neither inherently good nor bad; uncertainty just *is*.

Han and colleagues (2011) offer a panoramic view on diverse theoretical and empirical literature on uncertainty from different fields, psychology, communication research, nursing research, decision theory, risk management. They synthesize it in a taxonomy describing structure and terminology and a first sorting for the multifaced concept of uncertainty. As all taxonomies, it is organized in a tree structure. Uncertainty is at the head of the structure as a root concept, whose properties apply to all the other subgroups. However, they draw separate structures exploring three dimensions of uncertainty: *source, issue, and locus*. Uncertainty of *source* is subdivided into three types: Probability, Ambiguity, and Complexity. Ambiguity represents the lack of reliability or adequacy of information about probability; however, as Wayne and colleagues (2011) point out, ambiguity can emerge also from problems perceived as especially novel and complex, establishing a relationship with the third source of uncertainty, complexity. With this formulation, communication of uncertainty of risk and benefit of treatment limited to uncertainty about probabilities (Politi *et al.*, 2007) neglects other sources of uncertainty, ambiguity, and complexity. Timmermans, *et al.* show how exome sequencing to probe for a genetic cause of disease is discussed by laboratory scientists and clinicians. Their contending with, revising and revisioning the variants of uncertain significance, shows not only the emergence of new uncertainties and ambiguous causal relations but time as an important dimension.

The second dimension in the Han *et al.* taxonomy, *issue*, encompasses three categories — scientific, practice, and personal — including those issues identified in Kasper's taxonomy (2008). Uncertainty can arise in one of the three categories from the three sources of uncertainty (Probability, Ambiguity, and Complexity). The *issues* of uncertainty can be further subdivided into specific issues within which uncertainty can emerge. Specifically, scientific uncertainty involves the possible uncertainties emerging from diagnosis, prognosis, causal explanations, and treatment recommendations.[3] We report the tree-like structure in Fig. 2.2 providing some initial examples related to Mr Spencer's case. Practice uncertainty can emerge from the structures and processes of care; for example, uncertainty that can emerge in communication with a healthcare provider and between teams involved as information must be integrated within encompassing systems of understandings, intentions, ongoing action (Babrow, 1992,

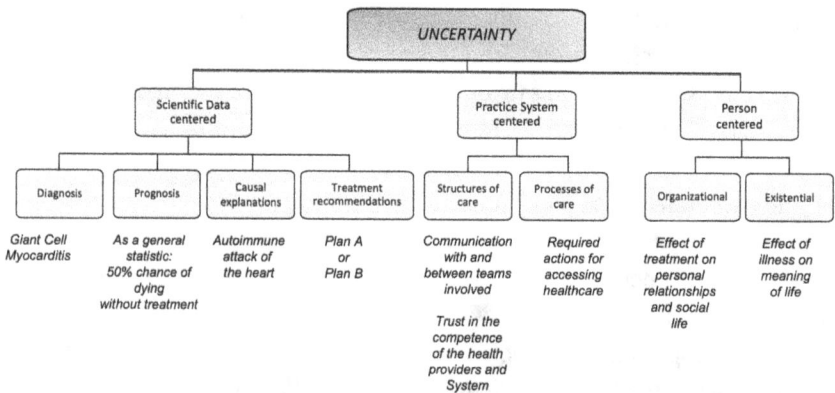

Figure 2.2: Taxonomy of uncertainty. Modified from Han *et al.* (2011). Note that Plan A and Plan B refer to Mr. Spencer's treatment recommendations. Plan A is medical treatment with immunosuppressants to restore his own heart's function while Plan B is Heart Tranplantation including mechanical pumps as bridge to transplantation.

---

[3]For an in-depth and critical discussion of how evidence based medicine from clinical trial outcomes frames and effects both the microlevel of clinical healthcare delivery and the macrolevel of healthcare policies and programs see the work of Aaron V. Cicourel (2011).

1995), and tolerance of uncertainty. Uncertainty also affects the person, as it can challenge one's entire sense of being, as in the case of patients and families facing the heart transplantation option. Han and colleagues further categorize *issues* of uncertainty into three main domains: data-centered, system-centered, and person-centered organized along a line from disease-centered to patient-centered. It is unclear what this line represents; it could symbolize a continuum in which different frameworks can develop or in which a different way of framing them could affect the handling of uncertainties. However, questions regarding new forms of uncertainties linking the different domains are posed by Timmermans and Angell (2001) who find that residents interpret EBM to fit their work practices: Those residents who consult literature and guidelines to get quick answers to clinical questions and those who critically evaluate the literature. In each case, EBM might generate new uncertainties due to how residents understand standardized knowledge and integrate it in their clinical practice.

The third dimension in the taxonomy of Han and colleagues, *locus*, clarifies that they consider uncertainty as a characteristic of the individual's mind, a mental state (e.g., patients, clinicians), It is similar to what Tannen and Wallat (1987) define as knowledge schema and contrary to what they state, agreement or discordance of knowledge schema in the doctor's and patient's mind does not make it a relational characteristic per se. Indeed, as we discussed earlier, we consider a process to be a relational when it develops in interactions. However, the great usefulness of a taxonomy as that of Han *et al.* is that it allows to create an inventory from an otherwise muddled mass.

We will come back to this taxonomy in Chapter 3 when we have followed Mr Spencer for a few days as his condition changes and new uncertainty emerges in the process of decision-making. There we discuss how it allows us to build on this first sorting by establishing relationships among the various domains within the relational context of the encounter (Raia & Deng 2015b) thereby emphasizing the relational nature of uncertainty, shaped by discursive (Babrow *et al.*, 1998) and interactional practices.

Research Methodology

Our work is part of an ongoing ethnographic–participatory research project studying the practices of teaching, learning, and patient care in an AdHF program in a large US university hospital (e.g., Raia, 2018, 2020; Raia *et al.*, 2020; Raia & Deng, 2015b; Raia & Smith, 2020) with more than 500 h of recorded medical encounters between healthcare professionals ($n > 25$) and patients ($n > 125$).

Participatory action research

Our collaboration started in 2009, when two of us, Federica Raia and Mario Deng, initiated a series of informal conversations around the issues of scientific and technological advancement in persons' lives, as seen in AdHF. These conversations were followed by exploratory interviews with Mario, followed by a more systematic collection of his patients' and their families' narratives about their experiences in AdHF. This initial work culminated in a collaboration with theater professionals Vanda Monaco, John Henry Davis, and Craig Lucas for the writing and staging of two theater plays. We initiated our collaboration as a Participatory Action Research (PAR) project, involving the practitioners (e.g., Mario) in the research process from the initial stages as participant coresearchers. Rooted in the work of Paulo Freire, PAR has been largely used in education research, however, is increasingly used in health research, most prominently in Public Health (Baum *et al.*, 2006).

From our perspectives and interests, as scientists, educators, and practitioners, participatory research is a powerful research approach because, along with those who study the practices from the "outside" (i.e., researchers), those whose practice is analyzed (i.e., doctors) also learn from the research. Learning about one's own practice, reflecting on it in collaboration with other practitioners and researchers in our sessions has been transformative for practitioners' own practices of medicine and transformative for the training of medical professionals from an apprenticeship model to a critical, reflective practice. Participatory research has also been an important research experience for Federica as a researcher supporting one of the tenets of Education Research: moving the research in directions enriched by questions most relevant to practice and anchoring it in what is relevant to stakeholders to better their care and teaching practices. At the same time, it has opened the possibility for the researcher, Federica, to learn about AdHF as a disease, read related textbooks and journal publications, attend international and national heart failure conferences, and follow hospital rounds. Most importantly, it has allowed her to learn from those inspiring individuals, the patients and their families, and from those who so tenaciously and compassionately care for them, the practitioners and practitioners in training.

We found that the richness of the medical practice in high-tech medicine cannot be understood by a single perspective of either the researcher or the practitioner *alone*. Each person (patient, family caregivers, healthcare professionals, and healthcare professionals in training) has a complementary role and brings a diverse perspective to the encounter. There is understanding about one's body (patient) and knowledge of the body of Other (healthcare professionals, family caregiver) that changes; there is knowledge of science and technology and its integration in the medical encounter; and there are the experiences of illness, disease, and care.

Starting with expert practitioners

Based on Federica's work, rather than utilizing an often used deficit model, focusing on practitioners' weaknesses and showing how practitioners deviate from an abstract model of optimum practice, we conceive learning as emerging from becoming familiar with the practices and by being inspired by something bigger than ourselves. Based on this stance, we focus on what is working well, from who is recognized as an expert practitioner by colleagues, patients, and families alike, and what counts as relevant practice by these practitioners. Our research hopes to be transformative for the participants and researchers and generative for creative learning environments for learners and professionals.

Studying medical expert practices "that work" has its difficulties. It requires capturing subtleties because what feels good is rarely "a punch in the face," it is rarely obvious. In addition, expert practitioners cannot describe what and how exactly they act because their way of practicing is like a second skin. From a phenomenological perspective, it is similar to asking to describe how we position the left foot turning a corner of 30 degrees left walking down a slope of 23 degrees. We cannot describe it, but we know; we just walk.

For example, when Federica first asked about his practice, Mario stated: "my practice is a RelationalAct, a relational presence in an act that appreciates the moment of the relationship as a privileged phenomenon, recursively integrating biological, psychological, and social level aspects within each encounter situation ... unfolds in the moment–to–moment interactions with patients" (Raia & Deng, 2016a). Mario's answer is too abstract to make sense of his practice. In the tradition of qualitative research, one would say he was telling but not showing it; that is, as a researcher, Federica wanted to show what the RelationalAct looks like in practice, what it means to care in the practice of AdHF.

Ethnomethodology (EM) informed approaches such as microethnography, multimodal microanalysis, and conversation analysis, paying particular attention to the moment-to-moment interaction are fundamental methods for the analysis of the "know-how," the instinctive skillful fluid mode of being (Dreyfus & Dreyfus, 1988; Raia, 2018).

Moment-to-moment interaction analysis

Studying the moment-to-moment interactions in the institutional setting of the hospital allows us to explore the AdHF practice, making visible not only *what* people do, but the *how* of the doing. EM informed approaches such as microethnography, multimodal microanalysis, and conversation analysis, pay particular attention to courses of action and the meaning-making by formal analysis of actual practice (Goodwin, 1994; Goodwin & Goodwin, 1997; Hall & Stevens, 2015; Heath, 1986; Heath & Luff, 2007; Heritage & Maynard, 2006; Streeck, 2017; Streeck & Mehus, 2005). A large body of work has been done in studying various medical practices (e.g., Beach, 1995, 2009, 2014; Gill & Robert, 2013; Goodwin, 2000a; Hall & Stevens, 2015; Heath, 1986; Heritage & Maynard, 2006; Hindmarsh & Pilnick, 2002; Llewellyn & Hindmarsh, 2010; Mishler, 1997; Mondada, 2011; Raia *et al.*, 2020; Raia & Smith, 2020; Stivers & Heritage, 2001). One of the pioneers, along with Candace West (1984), ten Ave (Ten Have, 1991), Paul Atkinson, and Christian Heath (1981) of EM informed methods of research in medical practice (for review see Gill & Robert, 2013) is Richard Frankel. Frankel (1983, 1984) studied recorded medical practices and was the first with his colleague Howard Beckman (Beckman *et al.*, 1990; Beckman & Frankel, 1994; Frankel & Beckman, 1982, 2017) to develop a video reviewing method to ground medical education in systematic research of actual medical encounters.

Through microanalysis of video- and audio recordings, EM informed approaches use methods of analysis of talk–in–interaction that reveal the dynamic and unfolding implications of communication. For example, in the high-tech practice of oncology, Alby, Zucchermaglio, and Baruzzo (2015) studied the informal conversations among hospital physicians sharing knowledge for diagnostic purposes in oncology. They show practices of decision-making that are more nuanced and complex than those informed by cognitivist perspectives representing such processes as a solo, rational, and unidirectional (e.g., Brun *et al.*, 1997; Li & Chapman, 2020). For example, they show that diagnosis is not done in isolation by the oncologist but develops as a practice of "joint interpretation" (p. 9) within an interdisciplinary team of specialist doctors, which also includes postponing the diagnostic decision. Sterponi and colleagues (2019) show the discursive strategies utilized by doctors and patients to coordinate and negotiate courses of action, and time and length of activities during oncology visits. These examples show how studying talk–in–interaction unveils relational organization and co-operation of human action (C. Goodwin, 2017).

Focusing on the action taken and resources mobilized in interactional situations to make sense of what it means to "understand" is common to all methods of talk-in-interaction (R. Hall & Stevens, 2015; Koschmann & LeBaron, 2002). Within sequences of talk-in-interaction, Goodwin (1994), for example, demonstrates that what distinguishes one profession from another is a professional vision, the practices used by members of each profession to "hold each other accountable for-and contest-the proper perception" (p. 628). Goodwin describes this process as a process that develops a professional vision within a community of practice of a specific discipline. In the learning sciences, Stevens and Hall (1998) show that learning to see with and through inscriptions and what practitioners "treat as properly visible and invisible" (p. 109) defines relevant practices in the development of a "disciplined perception."

Meaning-making and being a certain kind of practitioner

From the earlier discussion, it follows that the focus of EM informed approaches is the meaning-making that multiple participants manifest while involved in carrying out courses of action in concert with each other (Goodwin, 2000, p. 1492). The focus of EM is on the pragmatic, concrete, specific realities of the courses of action of meaning-making in the world. Developing an understanding of what to do is essential for making sense of the social and professional world inhabited. This approach treats epistemology — the relationship between the knower and knowledge and the intelligibility of pragmatic actions — as a discrete core issue. Yet, the ontological dimension of "learning as becoming" and "being a certain kind" of person or practitioner is left unanalyzed in EM as if it were unproblematic.

Raia (2018) demonstrates that inhabiting our actions and making sense of the world goes beyond an epistemological stance concerning what and how we know and what counts as knowledge of the specifics of any particular practice. It emerges from an ontological understanding of who we are and are becoming in a continuous process of making sense of the world we inhabit, learning to be who we are (Raia, 2018; Schatzki *et al.*, 2005), and caring for the Other (Raia, 2020). Through the lens of Relational Ontology and Phenomenology of Practice, a professional vision (Goodwin, 1994) is not understood solely as a professional epistemological understanding developed in a sociocultural and institutional context (i.e., AdHF). It is also fundamentally tied to our historically and temporally situated being-in-the-world. A different understanding of being *this person, this* kind of practitioner opens different ways in which things matter and in which one can be and act orienting toward others and recognizable ends. It manifests not only in what we can do as members of a professional practice, how we do it, and what is important to us. In this way, we do not arrive at a separation of our emotional responses — a disembodied sense of performing a role in the world.

We follow Raia (2018, 2020) and treat the epistemological issues as aspects of emergent ontological ones. Specifically, while we utilize EM informed methods to unpack the moment-to-moment medical interactions, we approach them through a Relational Ontology and Phenomenology of Practice (Raia 2018, 2020) interpretation of interactions: we focus on what practitioners attend to, what becomes relevant to them to call for action, and their comportment in making sense of situations and others in practice as a manifestation not only of participants' pragmatic actions of meaning-making, but what matters to the participant, what a participant notices in practice to care for the Other (Raia & Smith, 2020). These together show in practice how the existential demand of being one*self* manifests.

Ethnographic approach

As Cicourel (1987) shows, in research on interactions in institutional contexts such as those within medical settings, the context within which the interactions need to be understood is given by the ethnographic fieldwork necessary to situate a stretch of talk within its broader institutional context. Federica has taken field notes throughout our project during medical rounds, encountering participants outside the hospital context, and collecting participants' oral and written narratives. We utilize these field notes and the clinical understanding to situate the medical interactions we encounter.

Iterative research model

We developed a research model that proceeds *iteratively* in three stages of data collection and analysis (Fig. 2.3). Each stage of the process with continuity of representation generates resources and structures necessary for the following stages to emerge.

Stage 1 — Encounter Recordings of AdHF encounters are longitudinally audio-/videotaped for 1 to (at the time of this writing) 10 years. We follow the encounters of a patient in AdHF, Mr Spencer, and his family with the AdHF team members on-call longitudinally.

The position of the tape recording is always documented to recognize the volume of different voices better and differentiate talk available to all

Relational*Act* Model

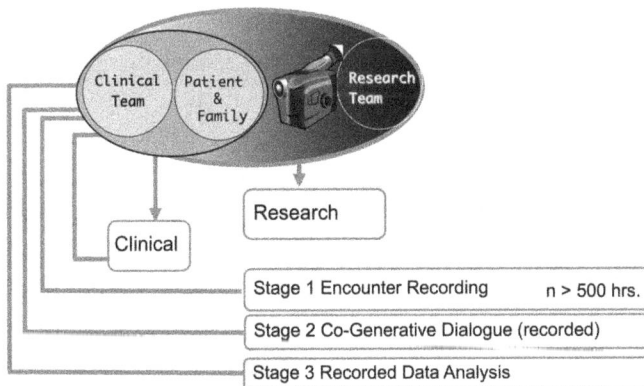

Figure 2.3: The Relational*Act* research model (Raia and Deng, 2015) is a participatory and iterative research model to study the AdHF practice. It proceeds iteratively in three stages of data collection and analysis; please refer to text for in depth description of each stage.

present in the room, which include patient and family (frontstage) or the discursive practices that, excluding the patient and family, involve only practitioners (backstage).

Backstage and frontstage: In his model of social interaction, the sociologist Erving Goffman (1959) utilizes the metaphor of a theatrical performance to make sense of how humans conduct themselves in social life. He argues that humans enact particular roles for others who, in turn, play the part of the audience. Goffman's model distinguishes the "frontstage" performance for an audience from a "backstage" behavior where an actor might be alone or hidden from the audience's view and hearing. In our work in medical interactions, unless expressly noted otherwise, we assign the role of the audience to Mr Spencer and his family. In frontstage, the shared region, the actions of the practitioners are visible to all, patient and family included. In backstage, the practitioners can refine their actions without being heard or seen by Mr Spencer and his family. Having always documented the position of the recorder allows us, as seen in Chapters 6 and 7, to distinguish such regions and make sense of the discursive practices.

Stage 2 — Co-generative dialoguing (cogen). Participating AdHF Attending cardiologist, AdHF Surgeon, and specialized bedside Nurse from the AdHF medical team, whose interactions were recorded in Stage 1, were invited to join weekly 2-h-long audio-/video-recording reviewing sessions as participant researchers. With them, the research team made sense of their taped practices and discussed the emerging elements and themes. Mr. Spencer and his family were also invited to participate and share their perceptions of the medical encounters. In our model, patients participate in no more than one or two sessions. This restriction is due to the interest in participating, barriers due to health conditions, time availability that can impede participation, and ethical concerns of intruding and possibly modifying healthcare professionals–patient relations in unpredictable ways.

The insights of those present on the scene richly inform the interpretation of the encounter from participants' perspective. Jointly reviewing the data in cogen sessions allows for a richer perspective on the practice, to address issues, to pose questions that are most relevant to practitioners and, as Sherin and van Es (2009) discuss, provides a window into what practitioners notice, including their interpretation of the taped activities and discursive practices. It also allows checking for the validity of the emerging patterns identified and interpretation of the data. As part of an iterative method for analysis, we watch each encounter in its entirety together, stopping the recording according to what each participant and researcher finds relevant or unclear. These "ethnographic chunks" (Jordan & Henderson, 1995) are then utilized to select similar events from other recorded encounters, which are then reviewed by the researchers (Stage 3). We follow up in subsequent cogen sessions, viewing and reviewing the events and discuss interpretations. Here, we report parts of these weekly reviewing sessions with the two participants and coauthors, Dr. D, the AdHF cardiologist who was the Attending on record during the recorded interaction in the Coronary Care Unit (CCU), and Dr. S, Mr Spencer's AdHF surgeon.

Stage 3 — Analysis of the practice recordings (Stage 1 and 2) is done to identify the resources (C. Goodwin, 2000b) utilized by participants as members to organize their conduct and reciprocal accountability as collectivity members (Garfinkel & Harvey Sacks, 1970). Events recognized as important in the emergence of themes, ranging from 30 s to 5 min, are transcribed utilizing a modified and streamlined version of the transcription systems elaborated by Gail Jefferson (Sacks *et al.*, 1974) shown in Table 2.1.

Table 2.1. Transcripts Symbols. We used a simplified version of the Jefferson's (2004) transcription system. Note that to avoid confusion, we have omitted punctuation symbols in the transcripts because, in the original Jeffersonian transcription system, they are used to mark intonational changes rather than grammatical symbols.

[	Left square bracket, on two successive lines with utterance by different speakers, marks the point at which the talk above is overlapped by the other talk a line below
=	Equal signs in pairs indicate that there is no discernable silence between the end of the first and the start of the following utterance, the first is '*latched*' to the following
—	A dash marks a sudden cut-off of the current sound
(0.5)	Number in parentheses indicates silence in seconds
:	Colons indicate that the sound that immediately precedes the colon has been sensibly prolonged or stretched
word	Bold and italic indicates some kind of stress or emphasis, which may be signalled by a change in pitch and/or amplitude
WORD	Capital letters indicate raised pitch or volume
(())	Double parentheses enclose comments by the transcriber
?	Intonation: A question mark indicates a rising contour
(hh)	indicates breathiness rather than laughter amid a word; in the cases included, it is near sobbing.

Microanalyses of body movements and prosody of the events are conducted on each event (C. Goodwin, 2000).

These events from Stage 1 and Stage 2 data include what a practitioner *notices* in cogen session reviewing the taped interactions (Stage 2) and *noticing in practice* events, those events in which collectivity members create and maintain a sense of what it is that is going on in the interactions as automatic rather than consciously chosen actions (Stage 1). As discussed by Raia and Smith (2020), cogen session data (Stage 2) provide a window into what practitioners reflect on and deem relevant for their own practice, including their interpretation of the videotaped activities. Analysis of Stage 1 taped data, as Heritage and Atkinson (1984) discuss, "enables repeated and detailed examination of particular events in interaction and hence greatly enhances the range and precision of the observations that can be made. The use of such materials has the additional advantage of providing hearers and, to a lesser extent, readers of research reports with direct access to the data about which analytic claims are being made, thereby making them available for public scrutiny in a way that further minimizes the influence of individual preconception" (p. 4). The analysis shows how health professionals care for others, i.e., as said earlier, how the existential demand of being this doctor, one *self*, manifests in practice (Raia 2018), "in routine rather than consciously chosen actions notable for their unconscious, automatic, un-thought character" (Swilder, 2005, p. 84).

Our analysis is based on collections encompassing multiple encounters from our corpus. As argued by Schegloff (1987, p. 101), in single-case analysis, a range of phenomena from our larger corpus of "talk-in-interaction are brought to bear on the analytic explication of a single fragment of talk." Here, we present a single-case analysis (Lutfey & Maynard, 1998, p. 323) in which participant doctors are coresearchers and coauthors.

The data at various stages of interpretation is also presented in data sessions held in (1) the Co-operative Action Lab (CoAL), a weekly data lab composed of linguistic anthropologists, ethnomethodologists, conversation analysts, and science studies researchers and (2) the Care Learning and Becoming Lab (C_LaB), a weekly qualitative data analysis interest group composed of education researchers and medical practitioners. These meetings provide an additional research space to discuss methodological issues such as those presented by data transcriptions (Ochs, 1979) and the organization of segments.

CHAPTER 3
FRAMING THE OPTIONS

In Chapter 1, we followed Dr. D's discussion at the symposium and during his lecture to the Residents about the possibilities that Mr Spencer's preferences had opened to the healthcare providers on January 1. We did not explore how the situation unfolded because to make sense of what happened on January 1, we need to go back a few days to see how the relationships and communication patterns between Mr Spencer, his family, and the Advanced Heart Failure (AdHF) team develop. In this chapter, we go back to those days when Mr Spencer was hospitalized. We follow Mr Spencer and the AdHF team from December 24 until December 29 through Mr Spencer's diary excerpts, cogen excerpts, and the data from the moment-to-moment interactions with the medical team in the CCU.

The dialogue between Mr Spencer and the team unfolds in an uncertain and continually developing clinical situation during these days. Building on our discussion of *framing for the Other* and *uncertainty* in Chapter 2, we show how organizing different scenarios, possibilities, experiences in a meaningful context during the variable course of the disease in AdHF for a patient (*framing*) makes visible how *uncertainty* emerges and is negotiated in the moment-to-moment interactions as an integral part of the practice.

A Rollercoaster

Mr Spencer is hospitalized in the CCU with the diagnosis of Giant Cell Myocarditis. Within the last 2 weeks, he had two cardiac arrests; one due to lack of electrical activity in the heart (asystolic cardiac arrest); the second due to episodes of very fast but still regular heartbeats degenerating into lethal, rapid, and irregular heartbeats (ventricular tachyarrhythmia episodes degenerating into ventricular fibrillation). Mr Spencer recalls one of these experiences, describing his wife's face getting slowly into focus while he was regaining consciousness: her voice, first as a distant sound, becoming a closer and louder yelling, "don't you leave me! Keep your eyes open, STAY AWAKE HONEY! DON'T YOU LEAVE ME!"

Being in the CCU is a constant reminder of this experience and the difficult choices patients and families face, as Mr Spencer recounts:

> *Segment 3.1.* Every patient in the CCU unit has serious heart issues, so I was not the only person going Code Blue[1] from time to time. The alarm and announcement occurred multiple times each day. 'Code Blue! Code Blue! [Hospital Name] 7619. Code Blue! Code Blue! [Hospital Name] 7619.' We would hear people running down the hall. One night it was in the room next door. For nearly an hour, we listened to the elevated voices calling out directives and continually re-announcing vital numbers. The frantic activity sent furniture or other heavy items crashing into the wall. The alarm and flashing lights continued for the duration. I grappled aloud with [wife's name] on how far do we go as Christians to scratch and claw at hanging on to this life when we know that this world is not our home. It weighed heavy on her when I expressed that I didn't want to be shocked and pounded and pumped incessantly like that.

During the last 12 days, to prevent his antibodies from attacking his heart and inducing ventricular tachyarrhythmia or, worse, ventricular fibrillation, Mr Spencer had four plasmapheresis treatments. These procedures "wash the blood" by removing plasma full of antibodies from the blood and replacing it with plasma components without antibodies. As per Guidelines Directed Medical Therapy (GDMT) for Giant Cell Myocarditis, Mr Spencer has also been treated with high doses of immunosuppressant medication (Menghini *et al.*, 1999). At the same time, the AdHF team, based on evidence-based medicine criteria, has initiated the evaluation process for

---

[1] Code blue is an emergency announcement over a hospital's public address system requiring a team of healthcare providers to rush to the specific location and begin immediate resuscitative efforts of a patient in cardiopulmonary arrest. The specific location is given by the room number which contains the room and the wing location. For example, in Mr Spencer's narrative "7" stands for the hospital floor, "6" for the location of the ward and "19" for the room number on that ward so that the practitioners know immediately the exact location of the emergency.

Heart Transplantation (HTx) as a backup plan. Later, Mr Spencer will recount about these days:

> *Segment 3.2.* It is interesting how one gradually begins to accept things one would have never accepted before. For years I had reflected on the passing of my grandparents and others and was fairly adamant that I never wanted to be on life support. I certainly would not have been amenable to the idea of a heart transplant. When it was my time to go, I just wanted to be let go. Of course, I always figured that would come in my 80's or 90's, not at the fresh age of 50.

As discussed in Chapter 2, the possibility of accepting the idea of HTx becomes possible when one is compelled to uncover one's body as made of substitutable parts. In this process, "my heart" then transforms into a malfunctioning or broken "tool" that cannot support my life (Raia & Deng, 2015b). Learning to accept "things he would have never accepted before" is now becoming part of Mr Spencer's life experience.

It is Christmas Eve afternoon. Mr Spencer and his brother are in Mr Spencer's CCU room when the AdHF cardiologist on call enters. He brings good news; the tests have shown some improvement in Mr Spencer's heart function. Mr Spencer recounts:

> *Segment 3.3.* He told us that I might actually prove to be one of the extremely rare GCM [Giant Cell Myocarditis] cases where the disease is actually turned back, and the native heart regains some strength. He actually asked if I wanted to take my name off the heart transplant list! When he walked out, both [brother's name] and I broke down in tears of joy, thanking God. That evening I could not hold back the tears. Tears of joy at the afternoon's good news. Tears of sadness at our family celebrating Christmas Eve in a hospital room. Tears of gratitude for the love, mercy, and faithfulness of our God.
>
> Later, I was getting ready for bed, and everyone had left the room except [wife's, daughter's, son's names], and my dad, when I had my third "Code Blue." The room started spinning, and I said, "something's happening! What's going on?" The Code Blue

alarm sounded, and staff filled the room. The head charge nurse yelled at me to "COUGH! COUGH HARD! COUGH HARD![2]" Again and again she yelled as she watched the monitor. I was in ventricular tachycardia (V-tach) again. I forced myself to cough as hard as I was able, over and over again, until eventually it broke. The beeps on the monitor immediately slowed to normal, the Code Blue alarm silenced, the dizziness left, and the room slowly emptied.

During the next few days, Mr Spencer's' heart function is closely monitored, hoping that it can recover with immunosuppressive therapy. Mr Spencer is worried. He just overheard a conversation among doctors of the General Cardiology (GC) team (primary team[3]) in hallways outside his room:

Segment 3.4. There are three levels of doctors: resident, fellow, and attending. The attending doctors are the veterans, the experts, the teachers. One of them appeared to be quizzing one of the [fellow (intermediate level) doctors on my case. "What do you think we should do?" he asked. "Get him a heart," she replied quick as a whistle. It sent a chill down my spine [...] Later in the day, I recounted what I had overheard to an attending doctor on my team [AdHF consult team] and let him know that I still wanted to do everything we could to keep my heart. He assured me that they would, but at the same time let me know that we definitely needed to keep moving ahead on the transplant end because it might become necessary.

---

[2]The evolutionary function of coughing is to clear the throat. As a side effect, a forceful rhythmic cough by means of compression and pressure changes of the thoracic and abdominal cavities provides effective blood flow through the body. In situations of ventricular tachycardia or fibrillation, this may assist in sustaining the circulation without direct chest compression. Thus, this mechanism of cough-assisted cardiopulmonary resuscitation constitutes a form of "cardiac massage" (LoMauro & Aliverti, 2018).

[3]When a patient is admitted to the hospital with a heart condition she or he is assigned to a primary team, a General Cardiology team, who is responsible for the overall coordination of care during the hospital stay, including admission, discharge, and coordination of all specialty consult services such as the AdHF.

Evidence-Based Reasoning

With Mr Spencer's health trajectory changing, the viable options also change. Figure 3.1 shows the estimated survival rate over a year for three options for a person in the condition of Mr Spencer on (a) December 23 and (b) December 29. On December 23, after completing four plasmapheresis

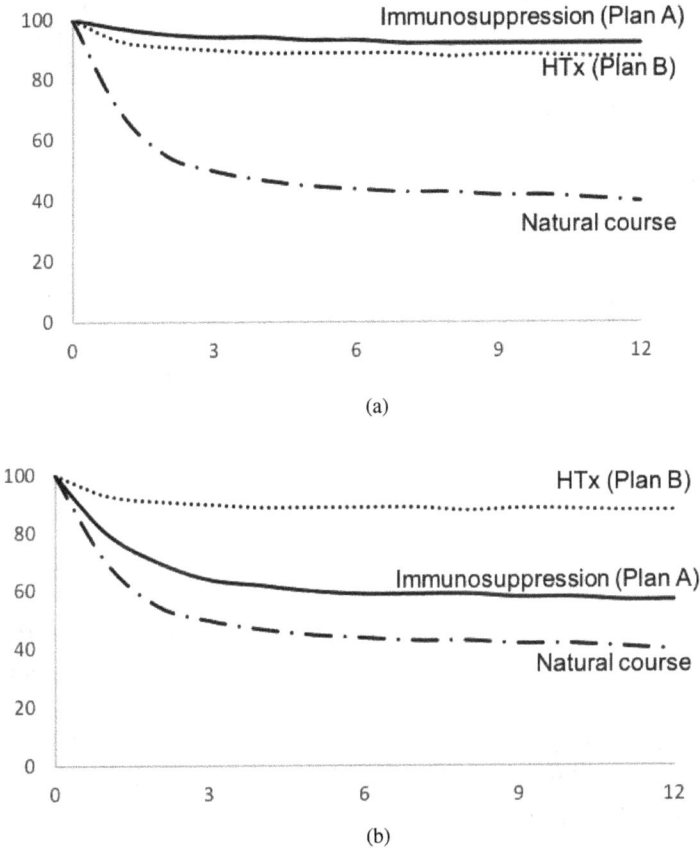

(a)

(b)

Figure 3.1: Evidence-based data of Giant Cell Myocarditis survival rates on Immunosuppression therapy, Heart Transplantation (HTx), and the natural course of the disease with no medical treatment (Natural course) (Cooper *et al.*, 1997; Elamm *et al.*, 2017; Lumish *et al.*, 2018). Please note that we labeled the curves Plan A and Plan B according to how the AdHF Cardiologist Attending, Dr. D, and Mr Spencer refer to the option of HTx and immunosuppression treatment, respectively, throughout their encounters. As discussed in the text, the two graphs (a) and (b) show the estimated survival for each option for a person in similar conditions as was Mr. Spencer on (a) Dec 23rd (b) on Dec 29th.

cycles and treated with immunosuppression, Mr Spencer's heart function stabilized. The continuation of plan A with immunosuppression treatment seemed, therefore, the best recommendation. It confers a higher survival probability than HTx, being less invasive than HTx and consequently associated with less risk.

Following the "code blue" on December 24, the team continually monitors and reassesses the situation. By December 28, Mr Spencer's heart function has not recovered, while the reappearance of arrhythmias worries the healthcare team. As shown in Fig. 3.1b, the continuation of plan A, i.e., immunosuppression therapy, may no longer be the best option for long-term survival. Plan B (HTx) may provide a better chance to reach this goal; the healthcare team needs to monitor the situation closely and, as Mr Spencer reported in segment 3.4, has initiated the evaluation for HTx. The GC Fellow's assessment is partly in line with this reasoning. However, evidence-based medicine, although necessary, is not sufficient for clinical practice (Braude, 2009; Cohen *et al.*, 2004; Feinstein & Horwitz, 1997; Goldenberg, 2006; Greenhalgh *et al.*, 2015; Henry *et al.*, 2007; Hjørland, 2011; Horwitz, 1996; McClimans & Slowther, 2016; Miles, 2009; Raia & Deng, 2015a; Timmermans & Mauck, 2005; Worrall, 2007). The GC Fellow's answer reduces any nuances of the clinical work, the possibilities, uncertainties, and experiences into "quick as a whistle" (Segment 3.4) certainties (Fox, 1957, 2003). Like other members of the AdHF team report,[4] encountering Mr Spencer requires understanding that he is a religious and spiritual person, inquisitive, and wary of any possible aggressive clinical action serving the sole purpose of prolonging the physical being. He strongly hopes to keep his heart (e.g., Segment 3.4). He has clearly expressed the desire to the healthcare teams to be actively involved in the decision-making process regarding his health and to include his family with whom he discusses and prays for each critical life decision.

Hearing the evaluation requested by a GC Attending and articulated outside his room by the GC Fellow disregards all that was known about Mr Spencer. The consequence of ignoring the person, Mr Spencer, while discussing the "case" outside Mr Spencer's room is that Mr Spencer starts questioning that the shared-decision-making process advocated by the

---

[4] See also Chapters 1 and 5.

AdHF team (Vucicevic *et al.*, 2018) will be respected and honored. He resolves to confront the issue by "letting" the AdHF Attending know that he still wanted to do everything possible to save his native heart. Mr Spencer, as a teacher first and currently as a school principal, is experienced and used to discuss, question, and lead. These practices act as particular resources, in Pierre Bourdieu's terms "capital" (Bourdieu, 1986), that Mr Spencer has access to. They affect his aspirations and expectations and affect the ability to negotiate and maneuver in the social space, what Bourdieu and Wacquant (1992) call "field" where he needs to contend the legitimacy of forms of medical authority in making decisions for his life. What would a person without such cultural capital and less used to debate and dispute have felt and done in this situation?

Framing from the Beginning

Dr. D had taken over the AdHF service (AdHF consult team) on December 26, two days after Mr Spencer's third code blue, and met Mr Spencer then. We did not tape the first three encounters between Mr Spencer and Dr. D.[5] However, 10 years of ethnographic work (including the study of recorded interactions) of this practice and Dr. D's description below can help us make sense of how he prepared and how the encounter developed. In a cogen session, Dr. D was asked to describe the preparation phase practice before meeting a patient in AdHF for the first time and before meeting Mr Spencer in particular.

> Dr. D: My experience tells me to be proactive in the very first meeting with patient and family. There are three things that I always do: first, I give them my business card so they can get in touch with me anytime, including calling my cellphone. Second, I sit down to talk with the patient and family.
> Third, I outline the scenarios . . .

Dr. D does not elaborate on the second step and moves to describe the third thing he does (reported below). However, ethnographic and micro-ethnographic work shows what Dr. D's "talk with the patient and family"

---

[5]For Institutional Review Board (IRB) compliance, we had to wait for Mr Spencer and his family to consent to our recording.

entails. In outpatient visits, e.g., Dr. D usually commences with questions that start from either something that he notices in the room, such as a symbol on the patient's T-shirt, which gives him a doorway into asking personal lifeworld questions, or from an issue contingent on the visit, for instance, how long it took to get to the hospital. He asks where the patient lives, how life is there, and then questions about the family and ways of life follow naturally. Dr. D proceeds by building on the answers received with follow-up questions or connecting what he is learning about the patient to his lifeworld events. It often follows that the patient and family ask lifeworld questions in return. The brief description Dr. D offers is consistent with the know-how, an instinctive skillful fluid mode of being (Dreyfus & Dreyfus, 1988) we have referred to in Chapter 2. Unless a problem forcing a person to enter a more deliberate mode emerges, this "know-how" becomes impossible to describe. It is doubtful that Dr. D had such interruptions when talking with the patient and family about their lifeworld. In comparison, the detailed account of Dr. D's third step in the first medical encounter seems to result from a deliberate practice built on experience.

Dr. D continues:

> Third, I outline the scenarios. I usually say just for the sake of completeness that it's worth talking about all the options that could theoretically come up. Most of them feel very theoretical, kind of a general picture, because they are not affecting the patient right now. But at the same time, talking about the potential scenarios in AdHF, one of which will eventually become the actual one, becomes part of the overall plan from the get-go. So, to come back later on to our first discussion is much more straightforward. It feels much better than to say, at a later stage, when things are getting into a downward spiral in a crisis mode: 'by the way, we now have to talk about another option' that a patient never heard of before [in context]. In contrast, I can tell the patient: 'as you recall, initially we had outlined the different options [e.g., from immunosuppressant therapy to heart transplantation via mechanical bridge]. Now we're coming back to them . . .' and that makes people feel, really, always hundred percent good."

FR: It establishes continuity.

Dr. D: Yes, in this way, the patient becomes familiar with these options and what happens between two encounters gets a baseline we can use for follow-up. In a hospital situation, there are many other practitioners interacting with the patient and family, including those in training [interns, residents, and fellows], and patients hear conversations about the different options in various ways. Since I have outlined in the beginning all possible options, the patient already can conceptualize all this together with me and in a framework that has been already established. So if something gets said in a strange way by, let's say, by a junior team member, or has been heard by the patient as a fragment of a conversation among practitioners outside the room, the patient knows he or she can always follow up with me. So, in other words, to answer your question, and in the case of Mr. Spencer, framing our encounter from the beginning and outlining the scenarios together allows us to contextualize all that is coming not only during <u>our</u> upcoming encounters but also all the in-between encounters with other practitioners.

Dr. D here identifies the change in a patient's condition over time, including moments of crisis, situations when a junior team member misspeaks, or the patient overhears a fragment of a conversation among practitioners outside the room as problems, as possible reasons for his deliberate actions in outlining the scenarios. Dr. D's third step points to the importance he gives to *framing* the first encounter. All the possible scenarios are contextualized and perceptions organized so that all upcoming meetings, including those with other practitioners, enter the frame he builds with his patients.

In the high-tech medicine practice of AdHF, Dr. D discusses the need for framing during the first visit as fundamental for the patient to learn to frame and face the problems and various uncertainties, spanning from the ones related to medical science to the possibilities of different ways of setting up the options, e.g., having two equally possible plans, indicated in Fig. 3.1 as plan A and B. More specifically, Box 1 summarizes the process of evaluation for advanced therapeutic options. For Mr Spencer, Plan A consists of continued organ repair therapy (Option 1); Plan B consists of HTx (Option 3) and if needed machine implantation (Mechanical Circulatory Support [MCS], Option 2) as a bridge to HTx.

Framing allows addressing multiple issues, such as becoming familiar with a new complex life and medical journey and aspects of hospital practices. One of these is that Mr Spencer has reported overhearing an Attending General Cardiologist (GC) and GC Fellow discussion outside his room.

Mr Spencer comments on Dr. D's practice as follows:

Segment 3.5. Dr. D proved to be an incredibly personal and tuned-in doctor. From the first introduction he remembered all my family members' names.[6] He sincerely wanted to hear our concerns and apprehensions, took the time to answer all our questions, and always kept us well informed with each new development and options to be considered. Only when we had nothing more to ask would he start to leave, with a warm smile, and the words, "to be continued." With such a rare disease, and so many unknowns, here was a man who could speak knowledgeably and reassuringly about my diagnosis and possible approaches. What a blessing from God.

Dr. D's assessment of his practice of framing "that makes people feel, really, always a hundred percent good," and Mr Spencer's evaluation (Segment 3.5) are in agreement. As Mr Spencer reports, and as we have introduced in Chapter 2, framing the uncertainties for understanding the options promotes trust (Armstrong, 2018) because, as Kasper and colleagues (2008) show, it pertains to the sphere of uncertainty that can emerge from the patient's perception of the physician's competence and trustworthiness — which includes how risk information is provided and how the patient deciphers it.

We started this book with a quote from A Scientific Statement from the American Heart Association (Allen *et al.* 2012), and we have seen the perspective of the doctor and the patient. The questions we ask now are: how does it look in the moment-to-moment interactions of the encounter? Does Dr. D's practice of framing become visible in talk–in–interaction during the following days? How does framing support Mr Spencer through changes and new developments? To answer these questions, we need to turn to the data from the recorded interactions.

---

[6]Dr. D writes the names of family members and other important beings (e.g., dogs) in the life of the patients in the medical notes to make them available to all team members.

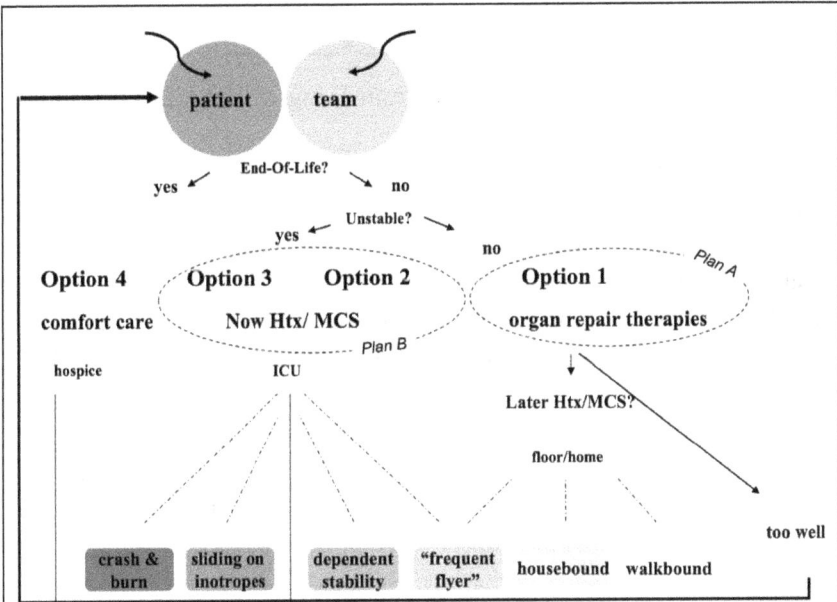

BOX 1: When a person develops Advanced Heart Failure (AdHF), often a referral is made from the treating general practitioner, internist, and cardiologist office/hospital team to a more specialized heart failure center team. An evaluation for advanced therapeutic options is initiated. These options may include — dependent on the patient's underlying condition — organ repair therapies, e.g. revascularization with coronary artery bypass surgery or stent implantation, unloading with aortic valve or mitral valve replacement, anti-arrhythmia therapy with ventricular tachycardia ablation (**Option 1**), heart support by Mechanical Circulatory Support (MCS), e.g. Left Ventricular Assist Device [LVAD] or Biventricular Assist Device therapy [BiVAD] (**Option 2**), heart replacement by Heart Transplantation (HTx) (**Option 3**) or quality-of-life (QOL) focused therapies, e.g. palliation care, comfort care or hospice care (**Option 4**). Options 2 and 3 are part of Plan B. The increasing severity of the heart failure syndrome is indicated by the boxes on the bottom of the figure from right to left, indicating "too well, walkbound, housebound, frequent flyer, dependent stability=stable on inotropic medication, sliding on

(*Continued*)

(Continued)

inotropes, crash & burn" (adapted from Deng & Naka 2007, Raia & Deng 2015b, details see text) is made.

The team's recommendation is based on the scientific evidence and the patient's values-based preferences. The recommendation involves an iterative shared decision-making process over time. The recommendation by the team is based on the estimated comparative survival/quality of life benefit from the more active surgical/interventional therapy (S/IT) in comparison to continued guideline-directed medical therapy (GDMT). The size of the anticipated benefit is based on the estimated probability of short- and long-term outcomes comparing two options for THIS PATIENT AT THIS TIME. The inability to precisely predict outcomes such as 1-year survival constitutes one (among various) domain of uncertainty in the shared decision-making process.

Changing Conditions and Evolving Options

We enter Mr Spencer's room on December 29 where he is with his wife, and CCU Nurse N, who is adjusting the infusion stand (Fig. 3.2). Mr Spencer sits in the hospital bed, Dr. D stands next to him while discussing the results from the latest ultrasound and the recovery trajectory of Mr Spencer's heart. The GC Fellow and the AdHF Fellow, rounding with Dr. D today, are both in the room attentively following the conversation. The GC Fellow stands next to Dr. D while the AdHF Fellow remains between the door and the sink at the foot of Mr Spencer's bed.

Dr. D is talking:

```
1    Dr. D:    when uhm we were in with the team uhm
2              we uhm uh were talking about
3              from the update ultrasound (0.7)
4              it is not surprising that things aren't uhm (0.8)
5              in-quotation-mark
6              just turning around (0.8)
7              it's uhm from the overall condition
8              something that uhm (1.0) is u::h (1.2)
9              gonna-be? (0.4) cha:llenging
```

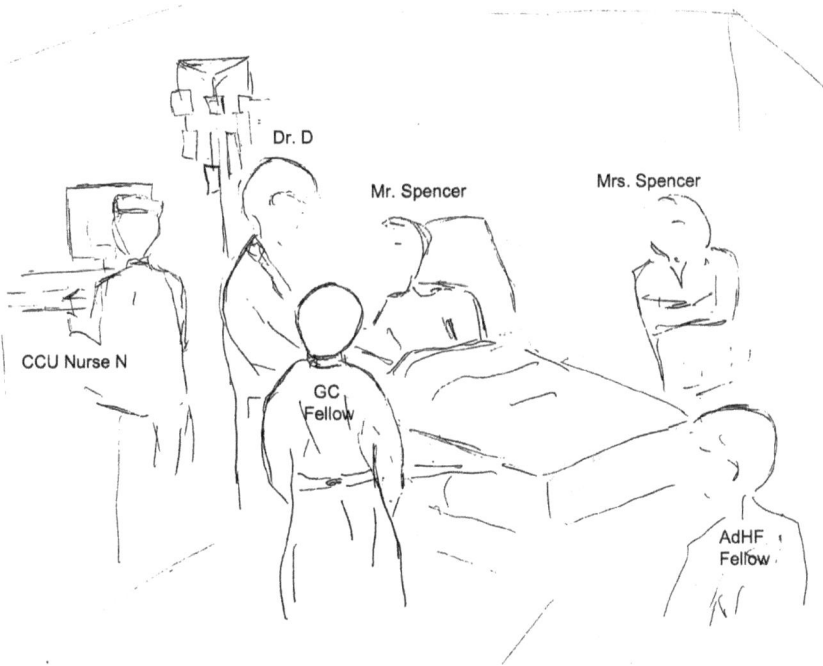

Figure 3.2: Mr Spencer's CCU hospital room. The recorder is on the shelf, behind Dr. D and Mr Spencer.

There is no possibility of recovering Mr Spencer's heart function. As the ultrasound results (line 3) show, things are not turning around (lines 4–6); the situation is challenging (line 9). Dr. D talks slowly with short acceleration on a few words (line 5) that seem to prepare for thinking carefully to what follows (line 6). His utterances are interspersed with hesitations ("uhm" lines 1, 2, 4, 7, and 8) suggestive of the talk's delicate nature (Silverman & Peräkylä, 1990). The slow but inexorable pace, the hesitations, and the number and the length of the notable silences (>0.4 sec) give the listener a sense that each of the following words is of utmost importance. Prominence is given to the utterance "not surprising" on line 4, emphasizing the syllables (bold italic in the transcript). The pause after a fast uttered "gonna-be" on line 9 also produces an effect of suspension marking, even more, the importance of what is uttered afterward: "cha:lleng*ing*." This is followed by another pause, marking the gravity of the situation: the possibility of recovering Mr Spencer's heart function is vanishing.

10	Dr. D:	we will be uhm (1.4) intensifying
11		the immunosuppressive therapy (0.8) uhm
12		and uhm (0.6) we will continue to (0.9)
13		closely monitor? (1.2)
14		uhm (1.4) but it's uhm
15		(0.5) ((swallows deeply)) (0.4)
16		even in the b:est (.) possible scenario
17		(1.2) that we
18		as we said yesterday hum
19		are uhm observing since you ca:me
20		here and we started the therapy? (0.6)
21		it's going to be some ((clears his voice))
22		first of all long term immunosuppression
23		which is the least (1.0) of a problem
24		but there is still (0.6) even at best possible immunosuppression
25		l:ong term uhmm some limitations in (.) good outcomes
26		in other words
27		this transplantation option
28		just needs (0.4) to be recommended
29		as a (.) close standby backup option (1.8)

Dr. D continues slowly to move toward the challenges ahead. He traces back a familiar step to Mr Spencer, the immunosuppressive therapy, then moves toward the challenges but not mentioning them yet (lines 14–16). Like a person, wanting to push a wheelbarrow through a rough, uneven, and unconsolidated terrain, needs to proceed with caution to create a path and moves back and forth to smooth and consolidate the soil, so does Dr. D. He moves in little increments, going back to familiar issues and then forth with hesitations (e.g., "uhm" line 14), swallowing so deeply that we hear his tongue snapping from having adhered to the palate (line 15). In silence or by clearing his voice (e.g., line 21), he pauses, pre-annunciating the importance of what is uttered next. What comes modifies what has been just uttered; the familiar immunosuppressive therapy, becomes long-term, the long-term therapy then becomes "the least of a problem" (line 23).

Dr. D's formulations do not include once the pronoun "you" to refer to Mr Spencer and specify for whom the situation is disappointing and challenging. He uses indirect pronouns and unspecified subject(s), e.g., it's, something, there (lines 4, 7, 8, 21, 24; 26–27) for whom there are a disappointment and long-term limitations in the outcomes. On line 19, the pronoun "you" refers to Mr Spencer but points to his arrival at the hospital.

After having reported about the team discussion, that Dr. D and the AdHF Fellows attended (lines 1–3), Dr. D uses the pronoun *"we"* in an ambiguous way (lines 17–20): "that *we (the team)*, as *we (you and I)* said yesterday hum are uhm observing since *you* came here and *we (can point to exclusive or inclusive)* started the therapy." English does not differentiate formally between exclusive and inclusive *we*. The lack of semantic distinction can point to a *we* used to include the patient, to mean *you and I*, or *you, me, and the team* or *we humans* or to exclude the patient, to mean *we the team* (Skelton *et al.*, 2002). With a return to the use of unspecified subjects (line 21), the third *we* (line 20) would be expected to be inclusive. The use of inclusive *we* is also consistent with how Dr. D reflects in cogen when outlining the scenarios (reported earlier).

Dr. D's involvement in the situation resembles neither the shared decision-making process of what to do next (Skelton *et al.*, 2002; Allen *et al.*, 2018; McIlvennan *et al.*, 2018), nor the process of minimizing resistance to reach consensus (Robertson *et al.*, 2011). While Maynard in pediatric consultations (Maynard, 1992) and in the articulation of bad news in general (Maynard 2003) finds that the clinician coimplicates verbally patient and family in the delivering of unfavorable diagnosis and bad news (e.g., by asking them to share their interpretation of symptoms), here we find that the clinicians achieve that nonverbally. Indeed, altogether lines 1 to 29, with a display of his emotional stance (M. H. Goodwin & C. Goodwin, 2000), point to the doctor's understanding of and participation in the patient's disappointment for his heart function worsening, and for the hope to retain his native heart vanishing.

30	Dr. D:	the (.) problem being
31		if for some reason we feel that things aren't heading the right direction
32		from that time point **on** to
33		transplantation
34		is not (1.0) an **hour** period
35		it's not (.) a **day** period
36		it's not necessarily a **week** period
37		it's not necessarily a **month** period
38		the median waiting time for heart transplantation
39		in this-region-of-the-United-States is three (.) point (.) zero (.) months
40		which i:s [hospital name]
41		which is the shortest in the country? for (.) population reasons (0.9)

Dr. D is at a very delicate point in the conversation. Introducing HTx as a very close option brings other complications. He continues slowly, moving toward the challenges ahead. Being approved for HTx requires waiting. The more hesitant talk on lines 10 to 25 for Mr Spencer's vanishing hope of recovering gives way to a reciting voice that takes the listener into a rising and falling rhythm repeated each line 34 to 37 to admit the only certainty. There will be a waiting time.

On line 40, we hear voices from outside the room approaching. The CCU Nurse N moves quickly but silently. She walks outside to talk to those who were about to enter. Dr. D continues slowly to move toward the challenges ahead. This is not the moment to interrupt him, and CCU Nurse N's monitoring and smoothly coordinated actions allows that.

42	Dr. D:	and that is why then
43		there may be this necessity of an additional bridge to transplantation
44		if that medication isn't stable enough
45		(1.0) talking about these pumps (1.0)
46		now (0.4) since we want to avoid at all
47		i:f that became necessary
48		a (.) *two* surgery situation (0.8)
49		the challenge for *us* is and
50		no one (.) is really-uhm perfect i:n predicting
51		the: (0.7) future likelihoods
52		you know if things are trending the wrong direction?
53		(0.5) then (0.4) have the active (0.5)
54		most active waiting list status ongoing
55		so there is a chance of things happening
56		in terms of transplantation
57		so that is the thought process
58		(3.0) ((clears his voice))
59		(6.0)

As we discussed earlier in Chapter 3, with an unsuccessful recompensation, i.e., with no heart function recovery confirmed by the latest ultrasound, the possible option of Plan B (HTx) includes the possibility of a bridge to transplantation via mechanical assist devices, if necessary. With Mr Spencer's worsening condition, the immunosuppressive therapy can no longer sustain Mr Spencer's native heart function. The waiting period for HTx can vary in time (lines 31–39) with a median of 3 months, Mr Spencer's heart will not support him for that long. This new development requires thinking more purposely about the scenario of a bridge to transplantation (line 43) by machine implantation. "These pumps" (line 45) are now looming on the horizon.

60	Mr. Spencer:	that makes (.) that makes (.) perfect sense to me
61		(5.0)
62		you're basically saying
63		go ahead and put me on the list (1.8)
64		and then (2.0) ((clears his voice))
65		the only question would be ((clears his voice))
66		I:f things came up earlier (1.2)
67		and we weren't really sure whether this heart (0.4)
68		was going (0.5) to make it or not
69		we have to make a split second decision=
70	Dr. D:	= that's brillia:nt thought (0.6)

For a person witnessing the dialogue, Dr. D's utterances such as "that is why then" (line 42) "talking about these pumps" (line 45), and "you know if things are trending the wrong direction" (line 52) would require an elaboration to be understood. Equally difficult to comprehend are the first lines 1 to 10 and all the references to the "list" to which Mr Spencer also refers (line 63). Mr Spencer's utterances, such as "if things come up earlier" (line 66), would require some elaboration for a casual witness to make sense of them; elaboration that we are providing based on ethnographic work. However, it makes perfect sense to both Dr. D and Mr Spencer, who have the sense of "what [it] is that's going on here" (Goffman, 1974). The two are continuing a conversation, as pointed out explicitly by Dr. D (lines 17–18), regarding the options framed during the first encounter by Dr. D.

With the disease's erratic behavior, Plan B now needs to be discussed in the frame within which the possibility of a bridge to transplantation with machine implantations is a viable option, if necessary. The reasoning of having Mr Spencer on the most urgent transplant list (lines 60–63) makes "perfect sense" to Mr Spencer. Dr. D does neither interject during the 5-s silence (line 61) at the end of Mr Spencer's statement of agreement (line 61) nor during Mr Spencer's numerous pauses. The 9-s silence at the end of Dr. D's talk (lines 58–59) is an open invitation for Mr Spencer to continue to talk after having introduced the transplantation option (Plan B). Dr. D's muted request is particularly noticeable because the silences on lines 61 and 63 are at the end of a finite statement and could signal Dr. D to take the turn and continue talking. However, he doesn't. An agreement to what makes "perfect sense" is not enough for Dr. D. Deciding to accept Plan B is an existential choice, and the gravity of what has been said needs to be fully grasped. To support Mr Spencer in making sense of it all, Dr. D needs to engage not only with Mr Spencer's thinking and learning about the disciplinary contexts (Campbell *et al.*, 2016; Luna, 2018; Richards *et al.*, 2020; Russ & Luna, 2013) of AdHF but, at the same time, to care for Mr Spencer (Raia, 2018, 2020), who is existentially shaken by the now very real possibility of losing his heart.

How Dr. D goes about it depends on what Mr Spencer will say next: "and then" (line 64), Mr Spencer's doubt emerges. The 2-s silence followed by the clearing of his voice emphasize what Mr Spencer utters next, "the only question" remaining (line 65), Mr Spencer clears his voice again. If the heart offer comes up too early (line 66), while there is still uncertainty on the chance that his heart could recover (67–68) . . . a "split-second decision" on a life-changing option must be made (line 69) to accept or not to accept the heart offer. Nuancing the discussion on making decisions within a much more complex context of uncertainty is a "brilliant thought" (line 70), replies Dr. D.

But, what about the bridge to transplantation through machine implantation Dr. D introduced before (line 43)? Dr. D follows Mr Spencer's lead. First to be discussed is "the split-second decision" uncertainty, a heart offer could come up "earlier" (line 66) when Mr Spencer's heart function could still be sufficiently stable (66–67). Paul Helft (2005), in communicating prognostic estimates of life expectancy in oncology, similarly reflects on the necessity for physicians to delay discussing a definitive, numerical prognostic estimate and embrace a style of communication that opens for patients the possibility to drive the flow of information. This necessity is more recently discussed in the field of ethical theory and practice by Emma Bullock (2016) who calls for a context-sensitive approach to medical disclosure.

Dealing with uncertainty

71   Dr. D: and identifying that as a problem is really important
72   because it's a very small chance? (1.4)
73   that we make (1.3) error number one type (0.6) which i:s
74   you have a heart transplant without needing it at that moment (3.8)
75   the question is how does it compare to error number two type (1.7)
76   meaning you (0.4) would have needed a transplant
77   but we came too late (1.8)

78		these are the only two (0.4)
79		*real* life practice errors that can happen (0.7)
80		if we make an error-optimally
81		we would have exActly the right time point (2.0)
82		like Ms. Moose had (0.6)
83	Mr Spencer:	mhm hm

Translating the evidence-based transition from Plan A to Plan B requires negotiating various uncertainties, including those inherent in any medical practice. Mr Spencer is listening as his acknowledgment (mhm hm) on line 83 indicates (M. H. Goodwin, 1980). Dr. D's response highlights the essential issues addressed in the literature of medical practice: the role that uncertainty plays in making sense of the complexity and ambiguity of health conditions (Fox, 1957, 2003; Timmermans & Angell, 2001b), available options and in the process of decision-making in general (Kasper *et al.*, 2008). Dr. D's response also brings to the fore the uncertainties and errors that can be made in "a split-second decision." Dr. D does not replace the uncertainty with an illusory certainty; instead, he frames it in the larger context of the disease's development and the available options to survive. The pattern of associating uncertainty with something familiar reappears, in this case, in the form of a possible positive and familiar outcome: "like Ms. Moose had" (line 82). Indeed, Mr Spencer and his family had contacted the Myocarditis Foundation after Mr Spencer was first diagnosed with Giant Cell Myocarditis. The foundation was created by a patient of Dr. D, Ms Moose, to help others struggling with this relatively rare but often-fatal illness; she had survived.

84	Dr. D:	but you know that's (.6) unpredictable (1.7)
85		we can just (0.2) fine tune
86		from the (.) continuous (0.3) te:am attention (.)
87		to (.) what's going on with you (0.5)
88		and you being completely informed
89		so it's not like oh
90		I have to think about this you know?
91		so that's that's that I want you to have
92		that mindset and everyone in the family
93		also so that
94		and Angel *((son))* comes up and says
95		wait a minute we have to think about this now
96		(3.7)

97	Mr Spencer:	we will talk about it today ((clears his throat))
98		I think (0.9)
99		I'm in agreement with *you?* (.8) h-yeah
100		we need to be ready (0.2) and uhm
101		if it was necessary only having one surgery
102		I understand it would be be:st
103		yeah we will disc-the whole family will be here (0.6)
104		and discu:ss that
105	Dr. D:	and if you like-uh I can you know 0(.6) come back
106		we can (1.3) uhm (0.9) discuss it together

Mr Spencer's questions

The last few lines 105 to 106 seem to point to a possible imminent exit of the doctor from Mr Spencer's room. However, Dr. D does not leave. He continues talking (lines omitted), commenting on the questions Mr Spencer's young daughter asked him the day before and connecting them to the main points of today's conversation — the continuation of immunosuppressive therapy and the expectation of HTx.

It is now that Mr Spencer returns (lines 115–116) to what Dr. D introduced as a possible option, a bridge to transplantation (line 43):

115	Mr. Spencer:	I have I have a question about (1.0) the-u:hm (.8) the (1.2)
116		assist (0.7) ((clears throat)) (0.6)
117		so really have a giant cell myocardhh (3.3)
118		for the rest of my life
119		whether I have a heart transplant or I keep my heart
120		I will be on immunosuppressants for this my life
121		and the potential of it coming back (0.4)
122		even in attacking a new heart or my own heart
123		if I keep *it*
124		is always there (0.6) right?
125	Dr. D:	uh-uh

As seen in lines 60 to 63 and 100 to 102, Mr Spencer expresses his agreement and summarizes his understanding. He has Giant Cell Myocard[itis], the end of the word is silenced by a sigh; silence; he will have to live with it for life (lines 117–118). He includes HTx as a possibility while maintaining open the option of keeping his heart (line 119). The hesitation in his speech produced by frequent quite long silences (lines 115–117) develops in slowly spoken utterances (lines 118–124), giving to each point: being on immunosuppressant therapy for all his life, with the potential risk of developing Giant Myocarditis again, even with a transplanted heart[7] — an existential gravity. Dr. D listens, assents (line 125), Mr Spencer continues to press his question about the mechanical assist devices whose names are still new to him (line 126):

126	Mr. Spencer:	((clears throat)) with a assist (1.3) pump (3.3)
127		the giant cell myocarditis it doesn't attack a pump
128	Dr. D:	that's a very good question
129		so if you had (0.7)
130		which is an option in general
131		a mechanical support device for lifetime (1.0)
132		that u:::h pump would not be affected by these white blood cells of yours
133		that are (.) so aggressive (1.7)
134		however since the pu:mp uhm i:::s a left ventricular assist device
135		that one that's for lifetime
136		the heartmate two like Dick Cheney had for eighteen months
137		you would ehm have to have
138		it's as*sist* device for the reason that
139		it assists your native heart to work (1.2)
140		not only the left side (.8) of the heart doing a little bit
141		along with the assist heart pump to the systemic ehm (0.5) circulation
142		but also the right side of the heart
143		would need to do a hundred percent of work
144		to get blood from the right to the-left-side
145		in other words
146		in order for that to wo:rk
147		we need to continue immunosuppression (1.3)
148		not for the *assis*t device but for the giant myocarditis
149		that still in your body (0.5) because your native heart's still in (0.9)

Dr. D responds first with an appreciation of the question (line 128). He restores the medical term mechanical support device (line 131) that repairs the colloquial term "pump" but does not exclude it (line 132). Mr Spencer's question is based on the reasoning that since the mechanical support device is not affected by his Giant Cell Myocarditis, he would need neither immunosuppression nor a HTx making the mechanical support device a long-term, maybe even lifetime solution. True, the disease does

---

[7]Please refer to Scott and colleagues work (Scott *et al.*, 2001) for a landmark paper that demonstrates that Giant Cell Myocarditis can recur after transplantation, fortunately, with a much better prognosis than without transplantation.

not attack a machine, however (line 134), since the mechanical support device is only assisting the native heart, which continues to contribute to the overall heart function, the native heart function needs to be preserved by continued immunosuppression because the Giant Cell Myocarditis is still in Mr Spencer's body (lines 148–149). With a left-sided heart pump, the left heart would have to do a little work, while the right heart would still have to do all its work "to get blood from the right to the left side" (line 144)

150	Dr. D:	a:nd th:*en* you had the situation that
151		being on a device that makes you (1.0)
152		I don't-wanna-say a bionic man (0.8) ((*smiley voice*))
153		but you know as someone who has hardware in the body (0.4)
154	Mr. Spencer:	yeah
155	Dr. D:	for a lifetime (0.4)
156	Mr. Spencer:	no [eh
157	Dr. D:	[**WHI**ch usually attracts microorgan:isms (1.0)
158		and then you have the immunosuppression going o:n (6.0)
159		an increased chance of opportunistic infections
160		which (0.9)
161	Mr. Spencer:	I know I got the=
162	Dr. D:	=make f*u*:ngi:, bacteria and viruses happy (1.0)
163	Mr. Spencer:	I don't
164		I got the answer to the question
165		we're not going to avoid the giant cell by a pump

As Dr. D discusses in cogen, Mr Spencer, in a last attempt to see his life without a heart transplant, is trying to understand whether a lifetime pump could be an option so that he can keep his own heart. Dr. D follows Mr Spencer's path and develops the image of how a "bionic man" (line 152) would be a suitable substrate for opportunistic infection. Note the overlaps (lines 156–157) and the latching (lines 161–162) of the two speakers' utterances. Mr Spencer tries to conclude, but Dr. D continues unraveling the uncertainties and difficulties of this solution depicting the "viruses, bacteria, and fungi" having a happy life in Mr Spencer's body with no opposition from his weakened immune system. An unpleasant vision that probably Mr Spencer would have preferred to avoid "I know, I got the" (line 161), "I don't" "I got the answer to the question: we're not going to avoid the giant cell by a pump" (lines 163–165).

166	GC Fellow:	uh-uh
167	Mr. Spencer	so the best options are (0.9) to keep this one or get a transplant
168		that would only be a bridge=
169	GC Fellow:	=mm-hmm
170	Mr. Spencer:	and a bridge we would hope to avoid
171		so yeah ok
172		that was hmm (0.9) [hmm
173	Dr. D:	[a good question
174		good question
175	Mr. Spencer:	the answer is very clear
176		((Loud beep sound, Dr. D is called))
177	Dr. D:	Dr. F ((to AdHF Fellow))
178	AdHF Fellow:	yeah, definitely

Mr Spencer "got the answer" to the question. He continues his reasoning regarding the next option on the horizon, a bridge to transplantation. The GC Fellow's sharp, fast, and high-pitch "uh-uh" (lines 166 and 169) seems to finalize an agreement. However, Mr Spencer continues with "a bridge we would like to avoid" (line 170) as to recall for the team the agreement that any possible aggressive clinical action that he would consider therapeutic obstinacy (e.g., Segment 3.4) should be avoided. "Good question, good question," recognizes Dr. D. Avoiding the bridge to transplantation remains uncertain. Is it needed? The question has no answer because the team does not know whether Mr Spencer will receive a heart offer before any further decline of his heart function. The team is preparing Mr Spencer for the eventuality. If needed, what type of bridge — artificial heart, Left-Ventricular Assist Device (LVAD), Left and Right-Ventricular Assist Devices (a Biventricular Assist Device, Bi-VAD)? The question has no answer yet. Dr. D has just started the conversation with Mr Spencer. We can infer here that the framing provided during the first encounter, as Dr. D discussed in cogen, does not include all details that could overwhelm a person who is learning about the new disciplinary context of AdHF, however, has been built to incorporate new information about the potential options in a cohesive form.

Dr. D's pager sounds loud in the room. He needs to leave the room momentarily (line 176) and calls upon the AdHF Fellow (line 177) to continue the discussion in his absence. We will continue following the development of this encounter in Chapter 4. Here, we want to pause to focus our discussion on the issues of uncertainty and framing for the Other we have introduced in Chapter 2 and seen emerging in the 9-min dialogue of this encounter (lines 1–176).

Framing Uncertainty: A First Discussion

As Mr Spencer describes (Segment 3.5), it is a *"blessing from God"* to be able, with his family, to confront the uncertainties together with his doctor. In the moment-to-moment interaction, we see how this happens. The talk, full of hesitations, rich in long and frequent silences, underlies the delicate nature of confronting various uncertainties. It gives space to all interlocutors to pace the delivery and receive information, express thoughts and doubts, and pose questions, integrating them within the persons' expectations, beliefs, desires, disappointments, and fears. Other relational acts similar to those reported by Raia (2020) engage the Other in a flow of events; e.g., Dr. D associates something familiar to the unknown and the uncertain to encounter, embrace, and negotiate uncertainties with Mr Spencer. Together with Mr Spencer, he gives a common pace to the conversation where playfulness and delays allow safely to inexorably proceed toward an understanding of what it is that is going on here. Indeed, it is within a process of *framing for the Other* that these relational acts conceivably promote the relationality necessary for trust to develop. Trust, rather than one of the subcategories in the tree-like taxonomy[8] (Han *et al.* 2011, 2019) shown in Fig. 2.2, becomes the substrate upon which the medical interactions between Dr. D and Mr Spencer and the AdHF team develop.

As we anticipated in Chapter 2, understanding the relationships among the various domains of uncertainty as they emerge and are negotiated in the discursive (Babrow *et al.*, 1998) and interactional practices requires us to consider the uncertainties as heterogeneous and multiplicitous parts of a web of relationships and mutual dependencies that change over time and with different situations. For example, Mr Spencer, during these days, is coming to terms with a profound existential and relational issue of living with the heart from somebody else, which opens hybrid spaces of existence located both inside and outside of his body. The relation with his wife is transforming

---

[8]One of the components in the taxonomy of uncertainty (Han *et al.*, 2011) is the *trust in the competence of the health provider(s)*, which includes how risk information is provided and how the patient deciphers it.

as well; she is becoming his caregiver, requiring both Mr and Ms Spencer to negotiate expectations, roles, and accountability. These transformations can give rise to coping strategies that enhance learning, partnerships, and high quality of life as well as create high levels of burden, anxiety, depression, associated long-term emotional consequences, and changes in quality of life for both patient and family caregiver creating an interpersonal conflict (e.g., Bohachick *et al.*, 2001; Bunzel *et al.*, 2007; Burker *et al.*, 2005; Canning *et al.*, 1996; Delgado *et al.*, 2015; Dew *et al.*, 1998, 2004; Ivarsson *et al.*, 2014; Marcuccilli *et al.*, 2014; Miyazaki *et al.*, 2010; Noonan *et al.*, 2018; Sadala *et al.*, 2013; Speice *et al.*, 2000).

At the same time, Mr Spencer is establishing new relations with each single AdHF team member, e.g., Dr. D, and with the team as a whole. As reported in segment 3.4, Mr Spencer's relation with the AdHF team "my team" establishes different accountabilities from those of the GC team. Indeed, Mr Spencer expects the AdHF team to be accountable for ensuring a shared-decision-making process, but not necessarily the GC team. When he overheard the GC team in agreement having him transplanted, without being part of that agreement, he reported it to an Attending doctor on his AdHF team. In the moment-to-moment interactions, we see these heterogeneous and multiple relations constantly emerging in the discourse (e.g., lines 1–20). Mr Spencer is also learning to inhabit a new world where scientific technologic advancements are integral parts, and medical science is often understood in the modern cultural paradigm of evidence-based science (Timmermans & Almeling, 2009). Evidence-based data is generated by large-scale research enterprise. Within this domain, the sources of uncertainty in the taxonomy of Han and colleagues (2011) — diagnosis, prognosis, causal explanation, and treatments — are translated into medical practice, with new emerging uncertainty. In other words, despite cutting-edge advancements in precision medicine, e.g., the molecular immunology–based precision prediction blood tests that may help reduce the prediction uncertainty in outcomes with AdHF (Deng, 2018), some uncertainty will remain and needs to be appropriately taken into consideration in the encounter. In Mr Spencer's case, immunosuppressant-based medical therapy and HTx outcomes are comparable for a person in the condition of Mr Spencer on December 23, as shown in Fig. 3.1a. The uncertainty reflects the risk for each option (Whitney *et al.*, 2004) and the time-dependent risk associated with either therapy. On a short timescale, an operation such as HTx is high risk compared to continued medical therapy (immunosuppressant therapy). However, on a longer time scale, HTx confers a lower risk beyond the perioperative period than continued immunosuppressant medical therapy. As Dr. D and Mr Spencer discuss, the Giant Cell Myocarditis disease has a continuous chance to flare up again, leading to the worsening of heart failure (lines 147–149), as was the case on December 24 to 28. In the medical interactions, Dr. D needs to translate large clinical trial results into a personalized treatment recommendation for *this* patient, Mr Spencer. The latter is skeptical regarding the potential futility of high-tech medicine.

As our discussion in Chapter 2 foregrounded, to nuance our under-standing of the medical interactions in this and Chapters 4, 5, 6 and 7, we need to include the uncertainty faced by the healthcare professionals originating from the different level scales at which uncertainties emerge. Mr Spencer's uncertainties about accepting the possibilities of undergoing HTx is expressed with the question on lines 66 to 68 when a heart offer can become available, and a "split-second decision" on a life-changing option must be made (line 69). Dr. D does not replace the uncertainty with an illusory certainty but points to other uncertainties as possible sources of two life-changing errors (lines 73–79): Mr Spencer receives a heart transplant without needing it at that moment, or Mr Spencer would have needed a heart transplant, but the team "came too late." Facing these uncertainties, the team needs to fine-tune and continue to monitor Mr Spencer's clinical situation (lines 84–85).

From the uncertainty related to the possibilities of undergoing HTx, others are generated; examples are those created by the required actions to access healthcare mediated by the institutional level: insurance approval, UNOS requirements for HTx listing, and its allocation system, as Dr. D discusses with Mr Spencer (lines 30–60). When arriving at a possible emotional and existential acceptance of a solution such as the option of HTx, other complications, risks, and uncertainties arise. Being approved for HTx requires waiting (lines 34–37), the only certainty.

Looking at the uncertainties in different domains as reported in Fig. 2.2 (Scientific Data-centered, Practice System-centered, and Person-centered) makes us speculate about the complex interrelation among level scales:

Medical science as a global level in which large-scale randomized clinical trials generate evidence-based data; Practice as a middle-level scale where healthcare providers and patient negotiate uncertainties in institutional contexts of medical care practices; and Person-level perspectives and experiences. However, these levels need not be thought of as structures, impermeable or independent from each other. Their relations are historical and changing over time. As Bruno Latour emphasizes, rather than "having to choose between the local and the global view, the notion of network allows us to think of a global entity — a highly connected one — which nevertheless remains continuously local [...]" (Latour, 1996, p. 372). Uncertainty, as a web of heterogeneous and multiplicitous relationships and mutual dependencies, requires a complex model of interactions with emergent properties of its own rather than a model with linear hierarchical connections such as the tree-like model.

Deleuze's and Guattari's "rhizomatic approach" to theory and research (1980) can be both an ontological and methodological approach to uncertainty. Like a rhizome, uncertainty is a complex system that ceaselessly establishes connections among things of different nature — e.g., Mr Spencer changing relations with his body with the heart of somebody else, with his family now caregivers, with his world, which needs to incorporate the world of scientific and technological advancement of AdHF. Like a rhizome, uncertainty is a system of various multiple and heterogenous relations that can change over time and with different situations transforming connectivity and meaning.

Considering uncertainty to have a rhizomatic character allows us to see that it grows following different paths and creating new connections stemming from temporary nodes. In this chapter, e.g., the temporary node, the uncertainty confronting the possibilities of undergoing HTx — from all the stakeholders involved — generate other uncertainties we highlighted. Methodologically, we can "enter" at any point in the "rhizome of uncertainty" and can follow Latour (Latour, 1996) in trailing how a node "becomes strategic through the number of connections it commands, and how it loses its importance when losing its connections" (p. 372). However, we cannot trace the entire rhizome completely, because it has no end.

The advantage of considering uncertainty as rhizome in studying practices of care is that we can see that the physician centers his framing around it. Framing, necessary to share and confront uncertainty, rather than acting as a rigid frame imposed on a person, unfolds around the specific uncertainties of the medical situation in which Mr Spencer's expectations and existential queries emerge. It is here that we found those relational acts such as giving time, with silences and repetitions, by waiting for Mr Spencer's doubts to be vocalized (as seen in line 66). To do so requires the understanding that it is not only by attending to Mr Spencer's thinking or his intellectual understanding but by caring for Mr Spencer (Raia, 2018, 2020) as a person who is existentially shaken by the very real possibility of losing his heart. When, in addition to attending to concept development and understanding, a professional needs to care for the Other (Raia, 2018, 2020), framing becomes *framing for and with the Other*, organizing for and with Mr Spencer the different scenarios, possibilities, experiences, course of the disease, and course of actions in AdHF for *this* patient, e.g., Mr Spencer, who has different knowledge, experiences, and worldview and in short time and under great existential distress attempts to make sense of it all. As Raia (2020) shows, for the physician, "supporting the Other to develop his path of being a patient in AdHF that is integrated with this person's lifeworld, gives meaning not only to what it means to care for others, but also to what it means to be an AdHF practitioner" (p. 16).

CHAPTER 4
INTERACTIONS WITH DOCTORS IN TRAINING

In Chapter 3, we left Mr Spencer's room at the moment when Dr. D's pager went off. Dr. D was guiding Mr Spencer through the implications that his worsening condition entails. The immunosuppressive therapy can no longer sustain Mr Spencer's native heart function. The option of heart transplantation is the most likely solution; however, given the uncertainties related to the timing of a possible heart offer and the Giant Cell Myocarditis's erratic behavior, a possibility of a bridge to transplantation needs to be discussed as a viable next step.

Before seeing Mr Spencer, as Dr. D shared with Mr Spencer (lines 1–10, Chapter 3), the team reviewed the most recent ultrasound. It showed that not only his left but also his right ventricular function is declining. Dr. D and the Advanced Heart Failure (AdHF) Fellow have discussed this development and the possibility of considering a bridge to transplantation via two mechanical pumps, one for each ventricle. The options vary from implanting a Total Artificial Heart (TAH) to one of the combinations of Left and Right Ventricular Assist Devices (LVAD and RVAD; a Biventricular Assist Device [BiVAD]) of different making and designs as we outlined in Chapter 3 (e.g., Paracorporeal Ventricular Assist Device [PVAD]-BiVAD; Heartware BiVAD). However, Dr. D did not address this developing issue before his pager went off.

With Dr. D leaving the room to answer the call, the social–institutional interactions in the room change. As Mr Spencer described in segment 3.4, "There are three levels of doctors: Resident, Fellow, and Attending. The Attending doctors are the veterans, the experts, the teachers," shaping a hierarchical organization of expertise. In this specific case, Dr. D is the AdHF cardiologist Attending, the AdHF Fellow is a cardiologist specializing in AdHF, and the General Cardiology (GC) Fellow is a general practitioner specializing in cardiology. When the Attending is paged and needs to leave the room, his role needs to be taken up by another doctor from the field of cardiology, and Dr. D chooses the next most experienced in the care of AdHF patients, the AdHF Fellow.

The process of becoming a professional, e.g., a general cardiologist, an AdHF cardiologist, in a community of practice, is a relevant part of the medical practice in teaching hospitals (Koschmann *et al.*, 2011; Raia, 2018; Raia & Smith, 2020). Here, practitioners are often engaged in a multiactivity practice in which concomitant activities: (1) advanced graduate medical education teaching and learning, and (2) patient care develop synchronously (Raia, 2018). Each activity has a purpose (to teach/to learn and to provide patient care), creating different possibilities of social positioning (e.g., being a learner/trainee, being a teacher, and being a healthcare practitioner) to emerge (p. 75). In the continuous engagement in multiactivity while becoming a general cardiologist, an AdHF cardiologist, trainees become accustomed to and are expected to step into a new role when necessary. In this case, they are immediately responsible for attending to patient care.

With this in mind, in the first part of this chapter, we focus on how each of the Fellows inhabits the new role. Specifically, we focus on how the AdHF Fellow takes up the role assigned to him by the Attending before leaving the room; how the GC Fellow partakes in the conversation now that the Attending is absent; and how the trainees take up their roles and partake in the interactions with one another and with the patient.

In the second part, when the Attending returns, we show how the conversation takes place during a process of decision-making.

Multiparty Conversation

Dr. D calls upon the AdHF Fellow (line 177) to continue the discussion in his absence.

177	Dr. D:	Dr. F *((to AdHF Fellow))*
178	AdHF Fellow:	yeah, definitely (.)
179		I did want to say that (2.2)
180		the right ventricle function is moderately to severely reduced *((Dr. D exits))*
181	GC Fellow:	reduced-to-severely-reduced?
182	AdHF Fellow:	yeah
183	Mr. Spencer:	so it's not just my left

The AdHF Fellow brings up the issue immediately, abridging the conversation into the looming possibility of an extra step before transplantation by implantation of not only one but two mechanical devices, each supporting one ventricle. This seems to be news to the GC Fellow, who asks for confirmation (line 181), and to Mr Spencer, who checks his understanding (line 183).

The conversation here turns into a multiparty verbal interaction, in which the designated speaker, AdHF Fellow, addresses Mr Spencer, and a third party, the GC Fellow, also intervenes. As more persons co-present in the room are involved in the production of the verbal exchange complexifying the discourse, it is helpful to recall Ervin Goffman's model of multiparty communication (Goffman, 1981).

Goffman considered the dyadic speaker–hearer communication model, which regards utterances as simple transmission, dichotomous and oversimplified. He conceptualized a more complex framework of social organization and involvement in discourse which distinguishes and nuances participants' role and participation at the moment of speech. For example, Goffman distinguished the participation of hearers into roles of ratified hearers (addressed and unaddressed recipients) and unratified hearers (bystanders and overhearers). In our case (lines 178–182), when the GC Fellow intervenes with a question, the AdHF Fellow responds directly to the GC Fellow (lines 181–182) as the new addressee before returning to address Mr Spencer. The GC Fellow who has not been directly addressed by the speaker, the AdHF Fellow, is recognized as a ratified hearer.

The AdHF Fellow's speaker role is similarly complex. Indeed, in relaying the message discussed with the AdHF Attending and the AdHF team, the AdHF Fellow speaks as part of a larger group (Goffman, 1981). In prioritizing the immediate delivery of the issue, the AdHF Fellow's mode of communication differs from that of the Attending. However, the AdHF Fellow delivers it by speaking slowly and with some silences within which his wording develops in conversation with Mr Spencer (lines 180, 184, 189; 198–199).

Overlaps and interruptions: Competition over care

The AdHF Fellow continues with an elongate s:o (line 184), indicating that the explanation to Mr Spencer's question (line 183) is pending (Bolden, 2009). However, the GC Fellow latches (=) into the talk and interrupts the AdHF Fellow. A quick "so" preludes the GC Fellow's explanation (line 185).

184	AdHF Fellow:	right (.) yeah (.) s:o=
185	GC Fellow:	=so the pumps would only be helping the left side
186		your right side would still have a hard time (1.9)
187		getting-enough-blood-flow-ac*ross* the *lu:*ngs
188		Ya:h
189	AdHF Fellow:	yeah so if you [uhm (2.3)
190	GC Fellow:	[ya
191		if you were (.) to require a pump at some point
192		you might need two pumps
193	AdHF Fellow:	one [for each side of the heart
194	GC Fellow:	[one for each side
195		mm-hm
196	AdHF Fellow:	[which
197	Mr. Spencer:	[not a great situation
198	AdHF Fellow:	yeah I mean it increases the complexity so (1.8) umh
199		you know it's good to (.) think (.) through these things=
200	GC Fellow:	=m-hm

From line 184 to 200, the GC Fellow operates several interruptions by latching to (lines 185, 200) and overlapping with (lines 189–190, 193–194, 196–197) the talk of the designated (line 177) speaker, the AdHF Fellow, with the result of taking the lead in the conversation with the patient moments later (lines 207–245). As observed during ethnographic work and discussed by the doctors reviewing the tapes in cogen sessions, this is not an unusual communication pattern. It seems to portray the competitive and self-profiling environment of academic medicine in general and the competition between the primary and the consulting teams, in this particular case, the GC team and the AdHF team, over the primacy of care for the patient.

There is no wheelbarrow carefully and cautiously pushed through rough, uneven, and unconsolidated terrain to create a path for Mr Spencer to work through the complexity and fear of what is happening to him, as seen in Dr. D's talk from lines 14 to 15. However, the AdHF Fellow, while trying to regain the floor as his right for conducting this activity (e.g., lines 189, 196), does neither interrupt the GC Fellow nor interject when the GC Fellow, searching for words, makes a relatively long silence on line 186, which, only in part, dissipates the mounting tension.

201	Mr. Spencer:	no I (1.3)
202		I don't need to think through that
203		I could see that picture

204		Okey
205		so that clearly answers that [question
206	GC Fellow:	[*BU*t it is

Mr Spencer moves to terminate the discussion about the BiVAD, by stating that he does not need to think through it, he has a clear picture, his question (line 183) has been answered (lines 201–205). As we will see below, Mr Spencer will have more questions, so it may be that the direct competition portrayed by the Fellows might not have been conducive to any further discussion at this time.

Creating Obstacles by Ignoring Uncertainties

The GC Fellow seems to interpret Mr Spencer's move to close the conversation with the Fellows as hesitation and indecisiveness in response to something that the doctor has outlined as necessary from an evidence-based algorithm perspective. Indeed, with a "BUT" uttered in a loud, high-pitched voice, the GC Fellow overlaps and contrasts Mr Spencer's statement and takes the lead in the conversation with the patient.

206	GC Fellow:	[*BU*t it is
207		an option if that if that does come up and we have *to*:?
208		it because you're the medications that you're on
209		aren't supporting your heart *enoughhh?*
210		and your other organs are *suffer*ing because of that?
211		That is always an option that we can go to
212		is putting in dual pumps if we had *to*
213		as a bridge to getcha higher on the *LIST:*?
214		for heart transplant to get it *fast*er also (0.8) okey?
215		so there are different ways that we can kind of uh
216		get you a little bit-higher-on the list if we needed **TO**

The GC Fellow entertains the case in which it is necessary "putting in the two pumps" (line 212) because the medications are not supporting Mr Spencer's heart *enoughhh* (line 209), and his organs are *suff*ering (line 210). Then, with questionable information (lines 213–216), the GC Fellow states that the team can get Mr Spencer higher on the heart transplantation *LIST* so to get, "it," a heart *faster.* As indicated in the transcripts, the Fellow stresses those emotional and salient words that impact Mr Spencer's life and medical trajectory. The stressed words highlight the importance of spoken information with the effect of guiding the interpretation. Indeed, as we see below, both Mrs Spencer (line 217) and Mr Spencer (lines 351–355) will inquire precisely about these issues.

The question mark (?) at the end of lines 207, 210, 213, and 214, indicates a pronounced high rising intonation. This way of talking, known as *uptalk*, turns each statement into a yes–no question, inviting listeners to assent, with a similar effect as adding "right?" or "you know?" to a sentence and preventing interruption by holding the floor with the suggestion that there is more to come (McLemore, 1991, 1992; Ritchart & Arvaniti, 2014; Warren, 2016). With the addition of informal expressions (e.g., organs that "suffer" rather than having a decline in their function "to getcha," line 213), the talk seem to infantilize Mr Spencer as an addressee.

The speech rate[1] (SR, measured in syllables per second), varying from fast (SR = 4.5) to very fast (SR = 6), when taking the floor (e.g., lines 224–225), is most conspicuous because comparatively much higher than that of the AdHF Fellow and the Attending (both ranging in the interval SR = 2.5–2.9). The GC Fellow's talk has virtually no pauses, no hesitancies, and leaves no possibility for any form of uncertainty to emerge. With the use of "we" referring to the medical team and excluding Mr Spencer, who is identified as an object of the medical team's actions (lines 211–212), the GC Fellow's talk transforms a process of making sense of the new options of a bridge to transplantation into an evidence-based algorithmic approach. It does neither require nor leave space for personalized shared decision-making.

217	Wife:	you say IF his organs start suffering
218	GC Fellow:	*m-hm*?
219	Wife:	[they're not suffering
220	GC Fellow:	[*no m-hm*
221	Wife:	[right now
222	GC Fellow:	[*no m-hm*

The clarification of and contention with the GC Fellow's speech comes in the form of a question posed by Mr Spencer's wife, "you said IF his organs are suffering, but they are not right now," that dissects the logic of the GC Fellow's reasoning. The GC Fellow's reaction is a series of loud and stressed

---

[1] SR is calculated as the number of syllables per seconds (Auer *et al.*, 1999; Rocco *et al.*, 2018). The count started with the first syllable uttered until the last syllable uttered in one turn of talk.

interjections *no m-hm no m-hm no m-hm*, overlapping Mrs Spencer's talk. They puncture the conversation like balls shot out of a tennis ball cannon. Listening to them feels like they are uttered with the function to prevent any uncertainty from emerging, quickly corking a bottle from which it is about to spill out. "Thankfully, the organs are not," the AdHF Fellow repairs (line 223), bringing an empathic ("thankfully") word to the talk, again interrupted by the GC Fellow who speaks now very fast as indicated by the dash between words (lines 224–225):

223	AdHF Fellow:	Thankfully they are [not
224	GC Fellow:	[because-the-medications-are-doing-their-job
225		and what-needs-to-be-done for your <u>heart</u>.
226		So it's working **enoughhh** to get blood flow
227		to all your other organs to perfuse everything-**but**
228		if we keep going up on those medications and your other organs
229		like your **ki**dneys or your <u>**li**</u>ver like that
230		start to s**uffer** because you're not getting enough blood flow to **them**
231		then that would be
232		at the time when we would think about
233		wanting to put in a device so that we don't (.) damage them further
234		**but** right now you're doing fine with them
235		and that's why we're going to keep you on thi:s
236		we're going to keep you where you are right **now** and
237		hopefully get you on **LI:st**
238		and we'll we'll go from it
239		we kind of take one day at a time and
240		always watching your numbers and
241		making sure that you're going in the right direction
242		or staying stable
243		oke:y. ((*sweet*))
244	Mr. Spencer:	okey
245	GC Fellow:	*oke:y.*
246	Mr. Spencer:	thank you
247	GC Fellow:	you're **ve**:ry welcome ehm
248		uhm here is Dr. D

The GC Fellow contextualizes the plan more clearly but forcefully, listing the organs that can still <u>suff</u>er but trying to balance that message by emphasizing that right now (line 234) Mr Spencer is doing fine with the medication. The GC Fellow reiterates the information, but the uncertainty is appearing in the possibility that the team can hopefully (line 237) get Mr Spencer on the **LI:st**; the only concern that the AdHF team does not have because Mr Spencer is an excellent candidate for heart transplantation.

Again, Mr Spencer is not included in the "we," which juxtaposes the team to Mr Spencer ("you"), reproposing the view of a team that acts on his body and Mr Spencer as an object of the medical team's activity. The interaction between the GC Fellow and Mr. Spencer and Mrs. Spencer makes visible how the GC Fellow's tacit and embodied understanding of clinical practice is anchored in scientific/medical authority as a particular kind of capital (Bourdieu, 1975). We see the GC Fellow using various discourse strategies to assert a truth, that of medicine. Viewed through a relational understanding of power (Alasuutari, 2018; Foucault, 1977), the GC Fellow aims to influence and control the discourse and Mr Spencer's and Mrs Spencer's understanding, conduct, and decisions. The called-up authority ("we, the team of the hospital") is embedded in the institutional and structural power that requires compliance (Meyer, 2010; Weber, 1978). Indeed, in cogen session, doctors and researchers alike reacted to the GC Fellow's talk describing it as having a patronizing tone, asserting "the power of medicine" over the patient's body, not a power to care for Mr Spencer as a person. A doctor who was not present on a previous cogen session when we listened and discussed this part of the encounter participated in a follow-up cogen session. Other doctors summarizing this part of the encounter used similar descriptors with the addition of "talking down to patient and family to the point of getting disrespectful." The doctor nodded: "oh yes, I know the type," which suggests that, unfortunately, this behavior is not that uncommon.

From line 243, the GC Fellow moves to close the conversation with a very softly and sweetly uttered oke:y, changing the previous prescriptive medical authority register. The "oke:y" with a flat final intonation also projects a contingent shift into closing the conversation that requires the addressee, Mr Spencer, and Mrs Spencer to agree. And they do. They surprisingly do. As we also see below, after having received such possible complications in Mr Spencer's clinical trajectory, it is unusual for Mr Spencer and his family to have no questions, no issues to discuss. Mr Spencer and Mrs Spencer collaborate in closing the conversation with the GC Fellow with the same closing token (line 244) and a "thank you" (line 246) finalizing the conversation.

However, the preparation for departure from Mr Spencer's room cannot be completed because this has to be done by the Attending, who has just reentered (line 248).

249	Dr. D:	sorry so you you just [talked about the right ventricular function [right?
250	GC Fellow:	[yeah [yeah
251	AdHF Fellow:	[yes
252	Dr. D:	[which which which which

Dr. D reenters the room communicating that he has followed, if not all, part of the conversation (line 249). Here, even though Dr. D was out of the room, he is not only considered a ratified hearer but, based on his rank as an Attending, can also take the lead in the conversation as soon as he reenters the room. Dr. D asks (line 249) to confirm what they have discussed in his absence and the GC Fellow overlaps twice with Dr. D's utterances. The GC Fellow's overlaps (line 250) have a different form now. With no move to take the floor they could be considered collaborative interjections (Beňuš *et al.*, 2011; Coates, 2013; Coates & Sutton-Spence, 2001; Edelsky, 1981). Indeed, as the Attending has the highest authority among the physicians and evaluates the GC Fellow's performance, it is likely that the GC Fellow would not take the floor. In addition, the GC Fellow has just closed the conversation with the patient and family caregiver and has nothing else to add and, as commented by other doctors in cogen, wants to "move on" to another patient in the CCU. The interjections have an overzealous character as if identifying which Fellow discussed the issue with the patient. However, Dr. D has left the AdHF Fellow in charge of the conversation, not the GC Fellow. Dr. D may be reacting to such zeal by filling potential silences with words to prevent being interrupted. He repeats the word "which" four times, an unusual repetition that we interpreted as asserting the right to speak for this activity.

253	Dr. D:	makes it even more important
254		and you talked about also what that *mean*s
255		*even if* we capture the trends and
256		*even if* you're listed on the highest urgency uhm status for transplantation
257		*and* uhm if the assist devices became necessary
258		it would be very well possible that
259		it would not only be left (0.7)
260		but potentially a bi (0.6) ventricular left and
261		right ventricular assist device (0.9)
262		and that is obviously a more complex assist device
263		we do have patients
264		you remember Ms. Airways
265		((turning to AdHF Fellow))
266		who went through exactly this
267		((turning back to Mr. Spencer))

268	I'm mentioning her name because she would be available
269	she and her husband
270	to talk like Mrs. Moose was in [city]
271	but in this case Mrs. Airways lives in [city] ((close by))
272	to talk about her experience when she came in with
273	giant cell myocarditis
274	she needed an assist device
275	all in two thousand eleven
276	in fall two thousand eleven
277	November two thousand eleven had a heart transplant
278	**a:nd** you should see her *NOWw* (1.2)
279	back to full time work you know
280	Ya-know
281	and so if you get interested
282	and we can talk about this later you know

Dr. D resumes the conversation by recapitulating the recent results on the right ventricular function and brings various layers of uncertainty to bear in the process of decision-making with Mr Spencer. Even with a well-developed plan B, the possibility of a BiVAD could be on the horizon. Dr. D commences three subsequent lines with the stressed words "even if" and "and" (lines 255–257), then with a suspension of any stress (line 257) continues starts two lines with same words "it would be," creating a rhythm to take Mr Spencer with him on a path to consider a BiVAD as a potentially viable option. Dr. D uses an intransitive verb (line 256) to point to a possible bridge to transplantation via assist device that prevents Mr Spencer from being viewed as a body, an object upon which doctors act. He talks slowly and again marks the relevant information and potentially existentially charged looming possibilities, e.g., line 259, with significant silences (lines 259, 260, and 261). The contrast with the GC Fellow's talk is stark.

As soon as he reintroduces to Mr Spencer the BiVAD (lines 260–261) as a "more complex device" (line 262) compared to a single (left) LVAD, Dr. D harnesses the experiences of other patients who suffered from Giant Cell Myocarditis: Mrs Moose, known to Mr Spencer, and Mrs Airways who had a BiVAD (line 266) implantation as a bridge to heart transplantation. "a:nd you should see her **NOWw** (1.2) she is back to work full time." Dr. D's voice is full of admiration and pride, communicated by a smiley voice, the stress of the word **a:nd** with the elongation of the sound (a:) as if a pivotal moment followed by the loud and stressed word **NOW**w, pronounced with a rising and then falling intonation on the elongated "w" sound. Mr Spencer can meet her anytime, she lives close to the hospital, and she is part of the successful AdHF patient support group initiated by the AdHF team: doctors, nurses, and social workers.

The BiVAD is discussed not only as a bridge to transplantation but also as a bridge from life inside to outside the hospital, opening for Mr Spencer a possibility of seeing a possible path outside his CCU room. Dr. D's construction of the bridge from inside the hospital to life outside is consistent with previous studies (Mattingly, 1998; Raia, 2020) showing how practitioners sketch out possible situations in which the patients can inhabit a life that is reconnected to what and to whom patients care about. In this case, the reference to Mrs Airways at work bridges Mr Spencer into the possibility of being back to his work, to which he is very devoted.

283	Dr. D:	so ventricular assist device
284		((turns to the Fellows)) thanks for mentioning that specifically
285		and so since we're talking in general
286		I just want to mention sometimes
287		a bi-ventricular assist device
288		if that's necessary
289		in the team will be compared against alternatively
290		to a total artificial heart (0.7) as a bridge to transplantation (0.4)
291		no::w: (0.4) that gets you [really to: (0.4)
292	Wife:	[as an option
293	Dr. D:	now since you have finished your breakfast ((smiley voice))
294		I thought it is a good time to [talk about the big picture
295	Wife:	[ah ah ah ah
296	Dr. D:	without (0.4) losing sight of a:ny (.) theoretical options

Dr. D resumes the conversation on the VADs: the BiVAD (line 283) and the TAH (290), indicating that he is building on what has been said in his absence (284). "No::w:" continues Dr. D talking to Mr Spencer (line 291), but Mr Spencer's wife overlaps his talk circumscribing the reintroduction of the TAH into "an option" (line 292). Dr. D recommences the sentence: "now" (line 293). He continues with a playful reference to Mr Spencer having finished his breakfast and ready for discussing the issue. He refers to the big picture (line 294), framing Mr Spencer's situation, as they have done together the first time they met.

297	Dr. D:	without (0.4) losing sight of a:ny (.) theoretical options
298		so the total artificial hear:t
299		would mean your heart would be

300	completely removed at that time (0.5)
301	and a artificial heart implanted (0.4)
302	and then you (.) would basically wait for the heart transplant with tha:t
303	and now people (.)
304	after first one-thousand-five-hundred total-artificial hearts-in the-world
305	the last ten-years
306	been (0.5) living with that
307	for two
308	three
309	four years (0.7) uhhhm
310	actually outside the hospital
311	but obviously had a lot of hardware in the *body* and (0.4)
312	the so-called freedom driver (0.4)
313	just imagine the (0.5) uherr
314	nice way of calling this eleven pound heavy (0.5) box
315	that you have to **carry** around with you
316	a f̲reedom **driver**
317	that is becau::se the previous generation was
318	a *big* washing ma*chine*
319	the big blu::e
320	you were kind of walking *after* the ma*chine* (2.0)
321	okeyehhh

Dr. D first describes the TAH, a machine that entirely substitutes a person's heart. Although playful in its content and delivery, the description is less than attractive for Mr Spencer, who is still hoping to retain his heart, who, as we saw in Chapter 3, could consider living with an assist device just to keep his own heart. With his move, Dr. D makes the BiVAD the less dreadful solution. It is not the first time we saw Dr. D engaging in this kind of move. In Chapter 3, we showed a similar move in response to Mr Spencer's hope to be on a LVAD to keep his heart and avoid transplantation. Then, Dr. D playfully depicted the "viruses, bacteria, and fungi" (line 162), Chapter 3 having a happy life in Mr Spencer's body with no opposition from his weakened immune system.

Reframing by Using Caring Power

Raia (forthcoming) has adapted the concept of "soft power" from its original use in international relations and foreign diplomacy studies (Nye, 2004, 2008) to describe the use of caring power in doctor–patient interactions. As originally defined in international relations and foreign diplomacy studies, soft power is used "to affect others to obtain the outcomes one wants through attraction rather than coercion or payment. A country's soft power rests on its resources of culture, values, and policies" (Nye, 2008, p. 94). In the context of caring for the Other, the power of enticing and attracting is not pointed toward desiring certain outcomes but to make therapeutic options familiar and accepted as possibilities. This adaptation of soft power into caring power can help us make sense of Dr. D's move. In caring for Mr Spencer, Dr. D needs to understand how to present new, unfamiliar, and often "scary" (Raia & Deng, 2015b) options to *this* person, Mr Spencer. The desired outcome for Dr. D is not to gain recognition of his or his team's cultural values — as it is for soft power — but for Mr Spencer to consider a BiVAD as a potentially viable option if necessary in his medical and existential journey. Dr. D knows that Mr Spencer will not accept a TAH, and Dr. D, making it an even less "attractive" perspective, points to it as a possible alternative. BiVAD is a more desirable solution!

As we discussed in Chapter 2, within a relational ontology framework, the existential demand of being one*self* manifests in what the physician is attending to, and his comportment in making sense of situations. These make visible what is relevant and matters to the physicians, what he notices while caring for the other, altogether giving meaning to what it means to be an AdHF practitioner and what it means to care for Mr Spencer. If we consider the two activities — patient care and Fellows' training — running at the same time in this encounter, repairing of the frame for Mr Spencer (patient care activity) is also a learning activity for the Fellows. On line 323, the GC Fellow is attending to the change and engages in the activity, which unfortunately also overlaps with Mr Spencer's talk.

322	Mr. Spencer:	[that's (.) gone
323	GC Fellow:	[so that's another option
324	Mr. Spencer:	that's gone a little too far
325	Dr. D:	*yes* (0.4)
326		so I would like to I just needed you
327		I'm sorry [though if that feels heavy [and intense
328	Mr Spencer:	[yah [yah
329	Dr. D:	but I needed (0.7) you to (.) kind of have a sense of
330		what's going through
331		let's say my mind or our minds right now (0.6)
332	Mr Spencer	there're limits in my mind (0.5) of uhm (1.2)
333		how far I'll go with this
334		and (.) that is at at the border
335		I don't think uhm (0.7)
336		I mean the *assist* to get to transplant (0.6)

337		I think (0.4) we've made that decision that if it's necessary
338		we would do *tha:t*
339	Dr. D:	yeah
340	Mr Spencer:	transplant if it was necessary to do that yeah
341		an artificial heart or anything that would require me to be
342		intubated (.) for (.) long periods of time
343		if I couldn't *eat* and *talk* (1.0) I don't wanna go that far (1.0) uhm (0.8)

Mr Spencer's change of characterization from line 202, "No, I don't need to think through that" a BiVAD he does not even name, to "the *assist* to get to transplant," (line 336) is the desirable outcome. Indeed, Mr Spencer does not even differentiate a single machine (LVAD) implantation from the possibility of having two machines, the BiVAD, implanted. Dr. D, who is also reporting what the entire team thinks, self-repairs (line 326) to express that he is sorry (line 327) that the discussion feels heavy and intense. The first step is done. Will this be the last step in the decision-making process? No. As we introduced in Chapter 1 (Allen *et al.*, 2012), and we continue to see in Chapters 5, 6 and 7, these are difficult decisions that threaten Mr Spencer's way of life, view of the world. Mr Spencer will need to let it be for now.

345	Mr. Spencer	Totally switching back to an earlier thing
346		two things actually (0.4)
347		one *is* (0.4) a *heart* (0.8) the transplant list (1.0)
348		id*eally* (0.8)
349		if I was going to get a transplant
350		we make this one last long enough so we only have one surgery
351		but if you *do that*
352		you ever really *rise?* to the top
353		I mean does the *pump* put you closer to the **top**?
354		if you don't put in a *pu*mp
355		do you ever actually *rise?* to the top of the list?

Mr Spencer "totally switches" the conversation. As we have seen in Chapter 3, when Dr. D feels that Mr Spencer is existentially shaken, Dr. D follows Mr Spencer's lead. Now Mr Spencer is confronted by the very real possibility of losing his heart and not only having to have one but two machines implanted as a bridge to transplantation. Mr Spencer needs to fully grasp it existentially, and Dr. D needs to start from what Mr Spencer will say next. Insisting on the topic of the BiVAD now will potentially lead to an undesirable outcome, as it did when Mr Spencer closed the conversation ("No, I don't need to think through that") with the Fellows. Mr Spencer needs to let it settle, and the doctor knows it.

As we anticipated, Mr Spencer inquires about the GC Fellow's two statements (lines 206–215): a dual pump "as a bridge to getcha higher on the *LIST:*?," and the team's power to get a heart *"faster.*[2]" Mr Spencer returns to the issue now that Dr. D is in the room:

356	Dr. D:	that's a good question in general
357		about the so-called allocation national allocation rule
358		uhm the fa:stest way (0.6) statistically speaking to have a heart transplant
359		i::s to d:o what could be done within
360		after team decision in place and if you agree uhm
361		within a mINUte and
362		that is actually since you already have this so-called
363		Swan Ganz catheter in place?
364		and one inotrope infusion?
365		there would be a second u:hm heart strengthening infusion added
366		and (1.0) uhm you would uhm (1.0)
367		assuming nothing else was there
368		and we had only the: in*fec*tion *que*stion to be finalized
369		you would be on the highest urgency waiting list
370		this so-called UNOS 1A list (0.6)
371		and as I said that's the
372		in this-region-of the-eleven-regions in the-United-States
373		the fastest way to have a heart transplant
374		the-highest-likelihood-to-have a transplant
375		*this* would *not* be*come faster* with a me*ch*anical *pu*mp in *pla*ce (0.6)
376		that *is* the highest (0.4) urgency-category
377		so you don't nee:d (0.4) a *pu*mp in order to (.) have a heart-f*aster*
378		I don't know if that answers that *que*stion
379	Mr. Spencer:	yeah it does

Dr. D starts with a supportive statement (line 356). Mr Spencer, if no infection supervenes, is a candidate for heart transplantation for the highest urgency waiting list, "the" (UNOS 1) "**LIST**." What about "the pump"? Dr. D's explanation is clear, not only in its content but in how it is uttered. Single words have their point of stress that guides the interpretation "*this* would *not* be*come faster* with a me*ch*anical *pu*mp in *pla*ce" (line 375). NOTE: With the US Allocation System Change effective October 18 2018 this system has changed.

Dr. D also repairs the GC Fellow's second assertion with "you don't nee:d (0.4) a *pu*mp in order to (.) have a heart-*faster*." Dr. D does not refer to any previous talk but does repair any possible misconception he expected

---

[2]The saliency of information carried out by these words is highlighted by the stress and high volume with which they are uttered.

was created or has overheard when he was outside the room. Mr Spencer, as we have seen in Chapter 3, summarizes his understanding and then thanks the doctor.

394	Mr. Spencer:	thank you so much
395		you know it's so good to (.8) like I said before
396		just to have the honest facts of what's going on
397		it helps make decisions and it helps my emotions to plan ahead (0.5)
398		I don't want to get more hopeful than is reasonable? (0.8) uhm (0.5)
399		but I don't want to get more dow::n (0.5) than is necessary to?
400		I just I want to know what's going on
401		and so I appreciate all the time you spend talking [with us
402	Dr. D:	[mm-hmm
403	Mr. Spencer:	it helps a lot
404	Dr. D:	mm-hmm it's a pleasure
405		and we'll be back

Dr. D and both the Fellows leave the room. "We will be back," the promise creates a sense of continuation, a conversation that continues, a relationship that builds.

CHAPTER 5

THE ITERATIVE NATURE OF DECISION-MAKING

In Chapter 4, we saw that caring for a person in Advanced Heart Failure (AdHF) requires understanding how the institutional power is used to frame new and unfamiliar options that can threaten a person's sense of being *this* person. As discussed in Chapter 2, in similar situations like the one Mr Spencer is facing, a person with AdHF, recognizing one's own body piecemealed into replaceable and substitutable parts and instruments, needs to contend with the threat to existence. The prospect of mechanical device implantation, of becoming "a scary character in the movie, half-man, half-machine," or "a science experiment" (Raia & Deng, 2015b, p. 136), intensifies the threat to one's existence.

In trying to dominate and even coerce Mr Spencer into accepting medical recommendations, the General Cardiology (GC) Fellow obtains three results: Mr Spencer ended the conversation, refusing to accept the recommendations, Dr. D needed to repair the possible damage to the respectful and trustful relations with the team, and the encounter extended for much longer than necessary. Utilizing the institutional power as a caring power opened the possibilities for Mr Spencer to start considering Plan B as a larger and more complex plan that includes a mechanical assist device as a bridge to transplantation and potentially viable option, if necessary. To achieve it, Dr. D needs to focus on *this* particular person, Mr Spencer, as a person who wants to be kept informed and be in the best position to understand and reason about treatment options and the development of the disease. It also requires understanding that Mr Spencer is not ready to inhabit the options of Plan B yet. As discussed in Chapter 3, framing for the Other requires to attend beyond Mr Spencer's and his family caregivers' thinking or *intellectual* understanding because framing is a process that develops and unfolds around Mr Spencer's expectations and *existential* understanding and queries.

In this chapter, we show how Dr. D builds on the original framing, transforming it with the changes in Mr Spencer's conditions during the following 3 days and helping Mr Spencer develop an acceptance for the options of Plan B. We report selections from the transcripts of each encounter that highlight the process and show a multiparty conversation.

Multiparty Perspectives — Building the Team

December 29, Afternoon

Dr. D enters Mr Spencer's CCU room while CCU Nurse N is giving the patient printouts of surgical consent forms Mr Spencer agreed to sign. Mr Spencer sees Dr. D entering and greets him (lines 4–6).

4	Mr Spencer:	doctor D
5	Dr. D:	hi
6	Mr Spencer:	how are you
7	Dr. D:	I'm fine I'm doing very *we:*ll (1.9)
8		and how is everyone *e:lse* here (1.0)

In addition to Mr Spencer and CCU Nurse N, there is another person in the room whom Dr. D does not know. Dr. D's question "how is everybody else" (line 8) is an invitation to introduce the new person. However, Mr Spencer answers by reporting on his stabilized condition.

9	Mr Spencer:	I think we're (0.7) back to
10		some stAbi:lity here *((smiley voice))*
11		looking forward to a (.)
12		better night's sleep tonight
13	Dr. D:	yeah (1.8)
14		that'll be a good thing to happen *((soft low key voice))*
15		I agree (0.8) *((very soft low key voice))*
16		okay

"We," Mr Spencer uses the inclusive "we" as he has done before (e.g., see Chapter 3), "we are back to some stAbi:lity" he utters with cheery excitement given by a smiley voice and variation of the volume and elongation of sound in the word "stability." Dr. D's assessment of the newly reached stability ("good thing to happen," line 14) does not extend beyond what Mr Spencer indicated, "a better night's sleep, tonight."

With a pivotal "okay" (Beach, 1993, 1995), Dr. D changes the topic. His response (lines 13–16) has two parts, it agrees to what Mr Spencer said and, at the same time, discourages thinking that it could be a sign of something else. When asked in cogen session, Dr. D confirmed this interpretation, sharing that, at that time, Mr Spencer had not yet abandoned the hope of saving his heart, which he found not surprising. Even if Mr Spencer has conceptually understood his medical situation, it does not mean that he has accepted it existentially. As discussed in Chapter 2, Mr Spencer and his family find themselves catapulted into a new world that is unfamiliar. Mr Spencer's historically and temporally situated being-in-the-world is a cohesive sense of been rooted in the past and projected in future possibilities of being the same person. However, with the dramatic and sudden changes in his life, this cohesion has been interrupted, disrupting his understanding, his sense of what matters, and his emotional investment in activities. As CCU Nurse N put it: "these are traumatic experiences for patients. It takes time to really make it sink," and it is upon the healthcare professional, as Virgil cared for Dante, to support patient and family developing a sense of the landscape where their journey is unfolding (Raia, 2020).

17	Mr Spencer:	rheumatologists were by
18		and shared a little bit of
19		your latest thinking about the
20	Dr. D:	like after we had this meeting after that
21	Mr Spencer:	yeah
22	Dr. D:	yeah good

The conversation between Mr Spencer and Dr. D turns to the family's latest encounter with the rheumatology team (lines 17–22), then his brother intervenes, asking Dr. D his last name.

23	Brother:	what was your last name again doctor
24	Dr. D:	D
25	Brother:	O:h okay
26	Dr. D:	So
27	Brother:	I have I have your uh
28	Dr. D:	you have my contact ((Dr. D gives the brother his card))
29	Brother:	no I don't (.) thank you
30		no I know about you
31		and I know you're much appreciated
32	Dr. D:	mhmm thanks ((softly uttered))
33	Brother:	so um but I I didn't have a facial connection
34		with the um with the name
35		so nice to meet you
36		I'm Rob and his brother (inaudible)
37	Dr. D:	I: ge:t it ((smiley voice))

Dr. D gives Mr Spencer's brother his business card (line 28), on which, in case there is a need to get in touch urgently, there is also his cellphone number. Mr Spencer's brother first comments on Dr. D as a doctor (lines 30–31); he explains why he did not recognize him (lines 33–34) and then introduces himself. Finally, Dr. D realizes too who is in the room (line 37).

38	CCU Nurse N:	his *vEry* devoted Brother:
39		who keeps a *vE:ry* close eye on him
40	Dr. D:	very good excellent
41	CCU Nurse N:	yeah he's got a very uh devoted family
42	Dr. D:	yes I think that's great

After Mr Spencer's brother has expressed appreciation for Dr. D, CCU Nurse N returns the praise with the specific acknowledgments of the brother's devotion and attentiveness (lines 38–41). By emphasizing the word *vE:ry* (line 39), the nurse simultaneously (1) reassures and alerts the doctor. Dr. D knows how inquisitive Mr Spencer and his wife are, and now he also knows that Mr Spencer's brother is equally inquisitive; (2) highlights the relevance of this moment. Mr Spencer's brother has been away and on his return today, as he also revels later in the encounter to Dr. D, has found his brother so much improved, maybe the immunosuppressant therapy is working! As Raia and Smith (2020) demonstrate, this kind of team communication, with one utterance carrying different meanings to different audiences in the room, is a highly sophisticated skill that healthcare practitioners learn in practice.

The conversation continues with Dr. D asking Mr Spencer's brother about him and his wife. It was them who found out about Mrs Moose (a patient of Dr. D) and who gave to Mr Spencer and his wife her book about surviving Giant Cell Myocarditis, becoming a heart recipient, and creating the Myocarditis Foundation.[1]

67	Dr. D:	Mhmm
68		and I think that's uh very helpful to (.) to have
69		other people's you know biographies on exactly this
70		so when she had her [Ms. Moose] heart transplant
71		which was October one two thousand and one (.)
72		at [Large Hospital name] so I was taking care of her

---

[1] Mrs. Moose was also referred to in Chapter 3.

Lines omitted

| 75 | Dr. D: | now was the same feeling |
| 76 | | that you're feeling right now you know |

Lines omitted

82	Dr. D:	she's {Ms. Moose] obviously back on the
83		you know transplant Olympics
84		golfing tennis and (.) all these things
85		so we started this myocarditis foundation

Lines omitted

89	Dr. D:	so it's just you know
90		back to life
91		and so that hh:hh is um important to (1.1)
92		get a feeling for but
93		the (0.6) momentary situation is um going through
94		these um (1.6) bumpy (1.9) moments

Dr. D engages in three subsequent actions: first, he builds on Mr Spencer's brother's story about talking to Ms Moose (lines 42–67, omitted). He acknowledges how helpful it is to have the opportunity to see how others have gone through similar medical and existential issues and, in doing so, addresses Mr Spencer directly (you, line 76). With these actions, Dr. D accomplishes two critical goals. He welcomes Mr Spencer's brother indicating that he knows how vital the brother's contribution has been, and reestablishes Mr Spencer as the addressee and a speaker. Mr Spencer is again the primary addressee and speaker in the multiparty conversation, adverting the possibility of becoming an object about whom participants talk. Then, with more silences in his talk, Dr. D addresses Mr Spencer's hope of regaining some stability (lines 9–10) by remarking that there are bumpy moments in the journey to transplantation (lines 93–94).

As Raia and Deng (2015b) show, initiating the medical encounter with an open question, such as "how is life," allows the patient to selects a preferred topic as the first subject in the conversation. Together with the medical and biographical records, the patient's choice of a first topic serves as a critical diagnostic tool assembled at the person level. Dr. D reintroduces Mr Spencer's first topic of hope to regain some stability at lines 93 to 94.

94	Mr Spencer:	we got a little bit of stability back this evening
95	Dr. D:	Yeah
96	Mr Spencer:	and uh we're um doctor R was saying
97		we're starting (2.0) Tac
98	Dr. D:	we added tacrolimus uh Prograf
99		uhm as an immunosuppression
100		next uh twelve hours

Mr Spencer will not have it; "we got a little bit of stability back this evening" (line 94). He moves to talk about the meeting with Dr. R, the rheumatologist Attending, and the immunosuppressant treatment to reverse Giant Cell Myocarditis. As he has done before, when Mr Spencer moves the conversation to a different topic, Dr. D follows Mr Spencer's lead. They talk about the effect of newly added immunosuppressant medication.

117	Brother:	here here's a question for you
118		that maybe (1.7) uh the rheumatologists
119		who talked about how
120		this drug focuses on T cells
121		as opposed to B cells and (1.28)
122		um (1.4) that (1.7) what is the theory of
123		how that would help (.) giant cell myocarditis

The conversation continues with a question asked by Mr Spencer's brother about the underlying immunological mechanism of Giant Cell Myocarditis and the related immunosuppressant strategies to reverse it. Dr. D gives a very detailed description, omitted here, of the mechanism and explanation for using the type of therapy. Questions asked by family caregivers are as important to answer as those questions asked by the patient. It is with family caregivers that the patient further discusses the therapeutic plan. Mr Spencer's wife and brother are the two designated family caregivers who will care for him through the treatment plan. As CCU Nurse N has indicated, Mr Spencer's brother "keeps a *very clo:se* eye on him" (line 39). While Dr. D sees the recovery of Mr Spencer's heart function as very unlikely, both Mr Spencer and his bother are hopeful for plan A — recovering Mr Spencer's heart function completely with immunosuppressant therapy. Indeed, Mr Spencer, referring to what Dr. D has previously said (line 100), asks when the new medication will be initiated:

| 219 | Mr Spencer: | when you sAy? within the next twelve hours (.9) |
| 220 | | are you talking about like |

221		tomorrow morning at five thirty
222		or are you talking about
223		before I go to bEd? tonight?
224	Dr. D:	yeah that uh the house team
225		we had discussed it during the dAy?
226		puts the orders in and
227		the next medication gets dispensed
228		so that's really that's why I'm saying
229		roughly you know yeah it does really
230		you know it'll be (.) in the next
231		twelve hour range with the next uh medications
232		I have to check maybe you had the first dose already

With "the house team...putting an order" (lines 224–226), Dr. D refers to the actions of medical residents who rotate in the GC team and are in charge of putting the orders in the electronic health record of medication, diagnostics, etc. The prescription can be prescribed directly by the GC team or by the AdHF team or other teams consulting with the GC Attending.

Dr. D responds (lines omitted) and immediately indicates that this is the same therapy prescribed after heart transplantation, reintroducing plan B and the issue of having to balance the overall immunosuppressant load with the possibility of elevated risk of opportunistic infection. He also refers to the Allomap test (Deng, 2021; Deng *et al.*, 2006) to monitor heart transplant rejection. Another attempt of reintroducing plan B. Another rejection: Mr Spencer recalls the conversation he and his brother had on Christmas Eve with another AdHF cardiologist Attending about some improvement in Mr Spencer's heart function that furthered the AdHF cardiology Attending to suggest some hope for Mr Spencer's full recovery (segment 3.3, Chapter 3). Mr Spencer asks:

306	Mr Spencer:	we were seeing a qUIETINg of the giant cell (1.9)
307		um does that (.) seem ((clears throat))
308		seem to be continuing? (.) that quieting or =
309	Dr. D:	= that's a good question
310		very good question (.6)
311		so for now *O:ver*all (.9) thi:ngs (.) seem stable (.)
312		so overa:ll we're in a (.5) you know
313		from the starting point (.7)
314		we would say (.8) best possible (.) scenario (1.3)
315		but um (.) having said that
316		I don't want this to sound like
317		everything is back to normal

318		you know (.5) in other words
319		among those scenarios that could be expected
320		it's the best expectable (1.)
321	Mr Spencer:	yeah
322	Dr. D:	but uh (.) that st*I*:ll may be let's say (1.3)
323		in the longer term not good en*ou*gh (1.0)

Dr. D responds immediately by latching (= line 309) to Mr Spencer's talk. Very good question. Oh yes, a very good question and Dr. D starts dampening down the expectation. Just as he has done in the morning, he talks slowly, treading through Mr Spencer's hope carefully with pauses and revoicing similar concepts until line 322. "But" he prepares, "st*I*:ll" the word is uttered with a stress, on a louder and longer sound of the "*I*," then the voice lowers again, and with a pause, Dr. D gives the final dampening to Mr Spencer's expectation with a future prognostication of long-term unfavorable outcomes. Mr Spencer's brother first and Mr Spencer subsequently quickly acknowledge that they are ready for both plan A and plan B. Dr. D leaves the room. Tomorrow morning they will meet again.

One could ask why Dr. D, rather than suggesting only plan B, does not say that there is no more hope for plan A. Mr Spencer has already agreed to plan B. He has signed the consent to be evaluated for heart transplantation and mechanical assist device implantation, and the process of listing him for heart transplantation is already ongoing. However, although the possibility of recovery is becoming less and less likely, there is no certainty yet. After the team recommends that Mr Spencer be placed on the United Network for Organ Sharing (UNOS) waiting list for heart transplantation, the team will have to consent Mr Spencer for the actual surgeries (transplantation and mechanical device). At that point, Mr Spencer will have to make a final decision to accept heart transplantation and/or mechanical device surgeries. If Mr Spencer is not ready to do such steps, he could decline.

Dr. D in cogen reflects on his "responsibility in providing Mr Spencer a space to make this existential decision at his own pace, as much as possible, working with his family, me, and the team through all the uncertainties and doubts within an unpredictable unfolding scenario. A premature answer would potentially destroy Mr Spencer's authentic embrace of plan B. I have to resist the temptation to take his nascent decision to accept it as a *fait-accompli*; it is not. I saw it happen before." In Mr Spencer's case, e.g., Mr Spencer could ponder that after all, "how far do we go as Christians to scratch and claw at hanging on to this life when we know that this world is not our home" (Segment 3.1). He could become suspicious of being pressured into accepting high-tech interventions that he is not sure would benefit him or could not agree with his values and his way of life. However, having framed the situation and the various options from the beginning allows Dr. D to return to the possibilities and options becoming more and more familiar to Mr Spencer rather than introducing new options with the development of the disease. As we anticipated at the opening of this book: "Advanced heart failure, with its high degree of prognostic uncertainty and complex trade-offs in the choice of medical care, demands a thoughtful approach to communication and decision-making. These interactions are not 1-time events but occur as an evolving series of discussions over time, particularly as a patient's condition changes. Such interactions may be difficult and time-consuming, and they often require planning to create a supportive environment for effective communication" (Allen *et al.*, 2012, p. 1939).

December 30

Mr Spencer's condition is stable, but, as Dr. D anticipated, there is no sign of his heart function's recovery. In preparation for today's encounter, Dr. D organized a conference call with a colleague from another university hospital, Dr. C, one of the leading experts in Giant Cell Myocarditis, to discuss the next step in Mr Spencer's treatment. It is with Dr. C that, over the last 20 years, Dr. D has shared and discussed the cases of Giant Cell Myocarditis. With Dr. C and Ms Moose, Dr. D had founded the Myocarditis Foundation.

In cogen session, Dr. D explains that inviting Dr. C to partake in the discussion of Mr Spencer's care has four main reasons. The first and most obvious is for Dr. D and the team to share their thoughts about Mr Spencer's condition and treatment with another expert. The second is creating a team teaching environment, in which everybody could participate in learning also from experts' discussion. The third is communicating to Mr Spencer and his family, to whom Dr. D will report the conversation with Dr. C, that the team has looked at all the different options and possibilities in light of current scientific data to know that all that was possible was done. The fourth is to maintain a culture of teamwork, dismantling or preventing the formation of a sense that a doctor acquires all the necessary knowledge with time and developed expertise. To learn that the ethics of caring for people requires, as Dr. D put it, "to jump over one's own kind of shadows, our medical egos."

Together, these four rationales build toward a global team concept (see also Alby *et al.*, 2015; Timmermans *et al.*, 2017) that includes other experts such as Dr. C and the patient and family members engaged in different ways and tasks.

When Dr. D enters the room on December 30, Mr Spencer is with his wife. Dr. D opens the encounter with his opening question: "How's life?" The question (line 3), as we discussed earlier, creates the possibility for Mr Spencer to select the preferred topic as the first subject in the medical conversation.

1	Dr. D:	hi everybody.
2	Mr Spencer:	hello (1.4)
3	Dr. D:	how's life? (2.6)
4	Mr Spencer:	another day of life (0.5), hanging on (1.6).
5		we are grateful for each day (3.2)
6	Dr. D:	I agree too (3.0)
7		It's actually a very (0.9)
8		good (.) general (.) concept (0.9)
9		in my opinion (0.5)
10		I like it (0.9)
11		why should it be different
12		for white coats who are rounding (0.7)
13		and for giant cell myocarditis patients, right?
14		cause honestly it's unlikely
15		that thousand years from now (0.9) umm
16		we'll be standing in this room? (.) and
17		discussing things (1.3)
18		although it's not completely predictable? (1.5)
19		but it's a good idea to be grateful for every day (1.0)
20	Mr Spencer:	I am (.)
21	Dr. D:	uhuh (2.5.)
22		okay how was your night?

Mr Spencer's answer (lines 4–5) invites Dr. D to comment on the one predictable fact that it is unlikely that thousand years from now they will be in the same room discussing things. With a playful take on uncertainty, "although it's not completely predictable" (line 18), he adds: "it's a good idea to be grateful for every day." Dr. D specifically reflected in cogen that he sees Mr Spencer and himself as two human beings confronting the inevitability of death as part of living.

The silence (line 21) did elicit neither further elaboration nor other thoughts or information from Mr Spencer. Dr. D then, with "okay" (line 22), marks the beginning of a new activity (Beach, 1993, 1995) and zooms in on the relevant event since their last visit the day prior, "how was your night?" (line 22).

```
23  Mr Spencer:  I slept good
24  Dr. D:       mm-hmm
25  Mr Spencer:  I uh (1.5) I felt (.) good energy
26               this morning after breakfast
27  Dr. D:       mm-hmm
```

Mr Spencer's first answer is positive. He slept well, woke up with good energy. Dr. D listens, his short "mm-hmm" (line 24, 27, 38) produced with falling-rising intonation, acts as a "continuer" (C. Goodwin, 1986, p. 213) treating Mr Spencer's prior talk as preliminary to further talk and, thus, encouraging him to elaborate on what he is reporting. Mr Spencer describes his last twenty-four hours (data omitted), which were okay, but:

```
37  Mr Spencer:  but uh (.) I took a wAlk
38  Dr. D:       mm-hmm
39  Mr Spencer:  and um (0.6) that kind of
40               zapped a little bit of my energy (.)
41               so I laid down for a while
42               and then I got up and ate lunch (.)
43               feeling pretty good again
```

The walk this morning "zapped" a little bit of his energy. Things got better after a nap and lunch. Dr. D inquiries about it.

```
44  Dr. D:       mhmm So how was this uh
45               when you took a walk
46               was(.) it was it like um muscles were (.)
47  Mr Spencer:  my muscles were [fine
48  Dr. D:                       [okay
49  Mr Spencer:  my legs were fine (.)
50  Dr. D:       uhhu (0.7)
```

Dr. D, as also observed in medical encounters in general medicine practices (Boyd & Heritage, 2006; Heritage, 2010; Mishler, 1984), solicits the expansion of this particular event. He specifically addresses or rules out a musculoskeletal contribution to the issue of the "zapped energy" (line 40) and invites (line 50) Mr Spencer to continue.

51	Mr Spencer:	I would feel (.)
52		we stopped about
53		four or five times (.)
54		mostly because in my head (0.7)
55		it wasn't dizzy
56		but (0.7) just (0.6)
57		things don't feel right in your head
58		you know
59		so we stopped (1.0)
60		let my heart catch up I guess
61	Dr. D:	mhm
62	Mr Spencer:	um (2.2) and so (0.7) I don't think I have
63		a huge reservoir of strength
64		so when you use it (1.4)
65		you use it and you feel it for a while
66		so
67	Dr. D:	[yeah.
68	Mr Spencer:	[I lay down for (.) what then
69		an hour or two?
70	Wife:	yeah
71	Mr Spencer:	and (1.0) after eating lunch (2.5)
72		I'm starting to feel (1.3)
73		pretty stable again
74		in the (.) stomach after eating lunch too
75		the (0.8) nausea in my stomach is (.)
76		kind of gone (0.6)
77	Dr. D:	okay
78	Mr Spencer:	so (1.7)
79	Dr. D:	good (1.0) very good (1.0)

Mr Spencer describes his walk and the difficulties he has encountered. The sentences in Mr Spencer's narrative "things did not feel right" (line 57), "we stopped to let my heart catch up" (line 59), and "I don't think I have a huge reservoir of strength" (line 63) alert Dr. D as signs of his progressive heart failure syndrome, lending the situation a sense of urgency. Dr. D does not interrupt the talk or interject during the long pauses (lines 59, 62, 64, 71, 72, 75, 78), further encouraging Mr Spencer's narrative making sense of what is happening to him and acknowledging these signs as a relevant part of the progression of the disease.

Dr. D promptly moves to the physical examination. After that, he recapitulates the discussion Mr Spencer had the day before with the infectious disease Attending, the content of which is also known to

Dr. D. Then, he summarizes the current state of medication, including the sets of immunosuppressants and prophylactic antivirals, antifungals, and antibacterials, all part of Mr Spencer's current treatment (lines omitted here). And, with a common and shared understanding laid down, Dr. D proceeds to describe his conference call with Dr. C.

129	Dr. D:	I had a talk a conversation
130		with my colleague Dr. C
131		this morning (.)
132		and since I also wanted the team
133		to participate
134		we had him on speakerphone
135		so everything you know
136		he's um an expert in myocarditis
137		as president of the myocarditis foundation
138		and uh (.) we had been in touch uh
139		also uh when I took care of Ms. Moose
140		because he and I've been working on this
141		in the nineties
142		so we are continuously in touch
143		in those situation where we want to
144		discuss if it's you know uh
145		and so we went through everything
146		uh that we're doing with you here (.)
147		and um (.) yeah
148		so that's uh the updates right now
149	Wife:	and the team is pretty much in agreement
150		with this
151	Dr. D:	mm-hmm yeah

Dr. D does not specify that the next step is moving from plan A to plan B (heart transplantation that includes the possibility of a bridge to transplantation via mechanical assist device). For Dr. D, there is really no hope left for plan A to be successful. He has brought plan B to the horizon numerous times during the last few days. However, as shown previously, while Mr Spencer and both his family caregivers, Mr Spencer's wife, and brother, have accepted the possibility to follow plan B, they are still hoping that plan A might be successful. Today, with the increased sense of urgency, it is time for Mr Spencer to come to terms with it. Dr. D, for now, leaves the topic undisclosed and hanging in the room to be discussed as soon as Mr and Mrs Spencer have no more questions on the current state, including team consensus about the current plan of treatment (line 149).

Questions, Ambiguities, and Explanations

As he has done in response to Mr Spencer's brother's questions the previous day, from line 173 to 220, Dr. D engages in a series of detailed explanations in response to Mrs Spencer's and Mr Spencer's questions. The specificity of the responses and the details increase with respect to the previous encounters with the family's and patient's increasing understanding and learning of the pathophysiology, prognosis, and treatment of AdHF. Below, we report the transcript with inscriptions to highlight the steps in the explanation process.

164	Wife:	and I haven't asked so
165		if you might be able to explain it to me (.)
166		but I was just curious why the:
167		why the medication that lowers blood pressure
168		when his blood pressure is already so low
169	Dr D:	that's a good question
170	Mr Spencer:	they changed that one though
171	Wife:	but you're still on one though, right? (.)
172	Dr D:	it's a very good question (1.0) um

Question 1
Apparent Contradiction

Mrs Spencer points to an apparent contradiction that brings to the fore the inherent ambiguity of translating evidence-based medicine and negotiating various uncertainties in medical practice. These include those uncertainties related to titration and the complex balancing of medications dosage to produce the desired effects and, at the same time, to reduce or eliminate the undesired ones. Dr. D takes a deep breath at line 173 and starts his explanation.

173	Dr D:	and on one **hand** (0.6) hhhm (0.7)
174		you want a certain blood pressure
175		in order to (1.0) u:h sustain your circulation
176		and perfuse all the organs
177		with oxygenated blood
178		on the other hand
179		if the heart is uh
180		the heart muscle is **weak** (0.8) um
181		you **nee:**d to (0.7) lowe:r the
182		re**si**stance against which the
183		heart muscle specifically talking about the left
184		but same on the right side of the heart
185		against which the heart muscle is **pump**ing
186		the lowering of blood pressure? i:s
187		one mechanism by **whi**ch the (.) re**si**stance
188		against which the heart is **pump**ing is decreased

Goal of Circulation

The response validates Mrs Spencer's observation; it does look contradictory. Dr. D continues, giving essential information, scientifically sound explanations, and why the team is pursuing this therapy. According to Dr. D's assessment in cogen, he needed to be completely attentive and have "to get it right" because Mr Spencer is suspicious of what modern medicine can do, and Mrs Spencer is worried about her husband who, while in the care of the team, is currently going through a very complex and life-threatening experience. The other participating physicians, in cogen session, expected the family to have a heightened awareness for the care Mr Spencer is receiving, which could manifest in scrutinizing the medication regimes while Mrs Spencer is becoming an advocate for the patient.

Dr. D's talk does not accelerate, but the fewer pauses give a more resolute tone. Stressing parts of those words necessary to make sense of the explanation, Dr. D starts with the need to have enough blood pressure to sustain the circulatory system, allowing the oxygenated blood to circulate through all the organs. If the heart muscle cannot pump strongly enough to provide oxygenated blood to all the organs, as Mr and Mrs Spencer know already, there are two possible solutions. As a last resort, they change the pump. Mr Spencer's heart can be substituted by a donor heart via transplantation or artificial pumps (mechanical assist devices). The less radical solution, if the situation stabilizes, is to treat the cause of the weakness like has been done so far, having Mr Spencer on a regimen of immunosuppressants to control the Giant Cell Myocarditis and support the heart muscle with strengthening medication to try to regain his heart pumping function. At the same time, to compensate for the weaker heart pump function, Mr Spencer is on high doses of vascular resistance lowering medications. These dilate his arteries, reducing the resistance against which the heart has to pump and allowing more blood to flow through to perfuse the organs with oxygenated blood.

189	and in a compensatory wa:y	
190	the: liters of blood pumped through the body per minute	
191	is *increased*	
192	so the mean blood pressure	
193	remains the same (.) but	
194	there may be (0.4) in other words	Transforming Mrs
195	*although* the um effect of those	Spencer's Question
196	medications is blood pressure *lowering* (.)	
197	because of the compensatory increase	
198	of uh (0.5) heart per*form*ance (.)	
199	the mean pressure remains the same	

The dilated arteries allow more blood to flow per minute, maintaining the blood pressure unchanged. But is a delicate balance, "a fine line to walk" (line 204).

200	Dr D:	*so* if a the blood pressure becomes too lo:w (0.4)
201		that is an indi*ca*tion and
202		you *feel* it as becoming *dizzy* that
203		we are (.) are dosing too high (0.9)
204		so that's something that is a *fine* **line** to wa*lk*
205		in other words uhm (0.7) we usually and
206		in general with heart failure situations
207		would say (0.5) then that the blood pressure level (0.4)
208		be it a hundred over sixty
209		you sometimes even you know
210		lower like ninety or something i:s not
211		ne*cess*arily *any* *pro*blem
212		*IF* you feel okay uh
213		because that's just indicating
214		the re*sist*ance against which
215		the heart is *pum*ping or
216		the workload against uh which it
217		has to bring up is optimized
218		but it's it's a fine line because
219		it must not on the other hand
220		be too low
		((sad voice))

"a fine line to walk"

Balancing Medication

If Mr Spencer feels okay (line 212), it means that the delicate balance is maintained. However, with the increasing weakening of the heart function, less and less blood can be pumped through the arteries and the blood pressure decreases, making Mr Spencer dizzy. Dr. D does not say this part explicitly, but his sentence (lines 219–220) is produced as if a deep sadness has quietly enveloped his vocal cords, marking the source of Mr Spencer's profound disappointment. This affective display goes beyond what Suchman *et al.* (1997) define as empathic communication in medical settings. Indeed, rather than a response to the "patients' attempts to introduce emotional concern" (p. 678) necessary to make the patient feel understood, it communicates a shared disappointment and, in turn, summons Mr Spencer's mood.

221	Wife:	it is running lower
222		than what it used to be
223		right?

Question 2

Confirmation

Mrs Spencer's second question highlights the issue of Mr Spencer's heart's function diminishing as the disease progresses. Dr. D reiterates the explanation:

```
226   Dr. D:    yeah (0.7)
227             so but that's essentially (0.5)
228             it has a lot to do uh with
229             how you fe:el in that situation (.)
230             it's uh it's really sometimes on the low side
231             but you're absolutely right (.)
232             it's something we have to watch it
233             the effect of (1.0) uh like milrino:ne? nipri:de?
234             are a:ll blood pressure lowering (0.4)
235             but not in an isolated way they have different
236             combined profiles (0.6)
237             and um the intention Is indeed
238             to (.) work towards um (.) lowering
239             the goal is not lowering
240             the blood pressure per-say
241             but what we call the vascular resistance
242             so it's something that
243             we have to just keeping (0.6)
244             and monitoring that the
245             blood pressure not too low (2.9)
```

Mr Spencer's heart function and the integrated circuits of the organs (organ-system level), his symptom presentation (body level), and his life-changing experience of having AdHF (person level) need to make sense in one cohesive perspective. Given as an initial framing, this cohesive perspective is addressed by answering Mrs and Mr Spencer's questions. Dr. D's task is to create a narrative in which *"I'm dizzy,"* low blood pressure, and the explanation *"I have advanced heart failure and immunosuppressant therapy may not be a good long term solution"* are in one framework to accept the next step. Mr Spencer responds:

```
246   Mr. Spencer:   I'm uh (1.6) would I be correct in saying?
247                  I'm stable
248                  but my heart doesn't appear to be
249                  getting any stronger? (0.7)
250   Dr. D:         yeah that's
251                  I think a good way of
252                  saying that right no:w. (1.3)
                        ((creaky voice))
```

253	Mr Spencer:	and (3.0) um (1.6) if that's the case
254		then we would probably look if
255		unless the heart started
256		to get stronger
257		we'd be looking more
258		towards transplant
259		right
260	Dr. D:	yeah (1.0)

After completion of Dr. D's explanation, Mr Spencer summarizes his situation. No plan A on the horizon; for the first time, all the questions he asks relate to having to live with plan B. It is no longer a possibility in case his heart would not recover, but the next step in his treatment. Mr Spencer asks (lines omitted) how walking regularly can optimize his fitness for the anticipated surgery and how long it will take to finalize the listing for transplantation. Dr. D summarizes all the steps in place and those that will need to be taken, such as getting "a clear" from the infection disease team.

302	Dr. D:	and (0.9) u::hm at the same time
303		as I said before
304		it's not like you're on the list
305		and then (0.4) imme:diat[ely
306	Mr Spencer	[I know
307	Dr. D:	and automatically we have to
308		do transplantation
309		but it's prepa:red (0.8)
310		also and (1.0) for everyone else who
311		wasn't here yesterday you know
312		also as a concept that (.) uh (.) you know
313		call it worst case scenario
314		on the list and the hearts not coming up
315		but the odds getting uh (.) uh sicker
316		then this mechanical pump concept (3.5)

Then Dr. D brings back the other options that are part of plan B, the pumps (line 316). He does so by reintroducing the uncertainty of the timing of receiving a heart and its unpredictable associated complications (line 315). Yes, Mr Spencer knows it; he overlaps with Dr. D (line 306). It is rare that Mr Spencer overlaps or interrupts the doctor. The only time we have found Mr Spencer overlapping the doctor's talk was during a discussion in which Mr Spencer hoped for the possibility of keeping his heart by accepting a mechanical assist device for a lifetime (December 29 morning, lines 161–162). Then, Dr. D described the "viruses, bacteria, and fungi" having a happy life in Mr Spencer's body with no opposition from his weakened immune system, a very unpleasant image. Mr Spencer tried to terminate that conversation, to shove off that image into oblivion. Our attention was captured by this overlapping pattern and interpreted similarly to lines 306 to 307 as Mr Spencer's signal to conclude the conversation on the topic.

Dr. D, as he has done in that case, continues talking. Indeed, an unusual move because the doctor generally listens carefully to Mr Spencer, does not interrupt him, and when he rarely overlaps, those tokens (hmm) function as continuers. The doctor's response shows no uptake of such invitation. Dr. D continues describing plan B as a complex and possibly multistep plan that always includes the possibility of a bridge to transplantation via mechanical assist device. As we see it reproposed throughout the encounters with Mr Spencer, Dr. D consistently describes plan B as a plan with multiple nonexclusive options. We interpret Dr. D's talk as an act of *framing* the path for Mr Spencer and, in cogen session, asked him to describe this moment: "I am worried that he [Mr. Spencer], now finally embracing heart transplantation as a possibility in his life, will consider, if medically necessary, the implantation of an assist devise as a step back that has the potential to overrule his commitment to the entire heart transplantation plan. A disappointment rather than a step in the right direction to have a happy, long life."

317	Mr. Spencer:	so if they list me on the list
318		is that just days away
319		or is that
320	Dr. D:	the listing itself is uh days away
321		the listing itself
322		that's that's something that is uh
323		basically everything major
324		that had uh to be completed is completed (7.8)

Mr Spencer does not engage in the discussion on mechanical assist devices but continues to inquiry about the UNOS transplantation listing process. Dr. D answers and then remains silent (line 324).

As discussed in Chapter 2, framing for the Other requires the doctor to attend not only to Mr Spencer's thinking and intellectual understanding. It requires caring for Mr Spencer (Raia, 2018, 2020), who is existentially shaken by a sudden life overturn and is living through a life-changing traumatic situation. Framing, therefore, is a process that develops and unfolds around Mr Spencer's expectations, understanding, and existential queries. In the moment-to-moment interaction, it is laminated by silences and repetitions. Silences create space for elaborating the meaning of what is going on in the person's life (e.g., line 324). Repetitions (e.g., lines 302–316) have the dual functions of pointing to what needs to become relevant, creating familiarity with new concepts and situations, and waiting for Mr Spencer's doubts and questions, indicating the pace of the progression toward new complexities. Indeed, as we have seen by his response during the encounter with the GC Fellow the day before (lines 206–248), Mr Spencer ends the conversation when pushed to accept a solution when not ready to do so.

In cogen session, the participating doctors discussed the possibility of having reached a closing moment for the encounter at line 324. The doctor has communicated the need to move to plan B, the patient agreed and asked appropriate practical questions showing that he understood. However, Dr. D does not conclude the encounter and remains silent, inviting Mr Spencer to speak. The silence hovers over the room like an unwanted thought. Will Mr Spencer feel comfortable talking about the bridge to transplantation now?

325	Mr. Spencer:	okay (.) my pacemaker is set at ninety
326		it was set at sixty before (.9)
327		and they set it up to ninety (1.4)
328		is that (1.7.) does that mean (.) that
329		my heart is getting weaker
330	Dr. D:	no: I wouldn't say that
		((creaky voice))
331		I mean the one consideration
332		is um (.) we you know the um (.)
333		one of the um situations
334		that happens with giant myocarditis is um
335		not only the (.) irregular fast heartbeat
336		but sometimes also (.7) a um slower (1.0) what
337		we call AV nodal block (1.5)
338		where it becomes a slow (.)
339		although it all the days that um
340		the last days it hasn't um happened (2.3)
341	Mr. Spencer:	so ninety is a fine place to be
342	Dr. D:	ninety is uh you know

343   it's an okay place to be (1.4)
344   so that um (.7) is in the range of
345   you know (.9) what it uh is good to be (2.2)

Definitely not. Mr Spencer, marking the beginning of a new activity with "okay," introduces a new topic, his pacemaker rate, which was increased from 60 to 90 beats per minute. Dr. D follows Mr Spencer's lead, as he has done before. Dr. D's talk continues in the same mode and style, giving no hints of surprise or disappointment in the introduction of a new topic that rejects, at least now, the discussion on ventricular assist devices.

After Dr. D concludes the explanation on the pacemaker, Mr Spencer continues, "there is one more thing" Mr Spencer clears his throat:

346   Mr. Spencer: um (1.1) one more thing
347   I (clears throat) um (1.7) when I'm sitting up
348   or if I'm lying on my side
349   Dr. D: mhmm
350   Mr. Spencer: this doesn't ever happen
351   but when I'm lying on my back
352   even if I'm in bed and I'm like reclined
353   Dr. D: mhmm
354   Mr. Spencer: I get these things where (.)
355   all of a sudden (.)
356   I feel (.8) um short of breath? and
357   a little cold and a little lightheaded? (1.7)
358   and if I lay on my side
359   it (.) tends not to happen
360   or when I'm sitting in the chair
361   it never happens
362   but when I'm laying on my back

Mr Spencer's inquiry on his new symptoms invites Dr. D to a subsequent in-depth explanation about the pathophysiology of AdHF, starting from the laying back as the typical position when "in heart failure, the shortness of breath becomes most pronounced" (transcripts omitted). It is a confirmation of the diagnosis of AdHF and, as Mr and Mrs Spencer know, the necessity to proceed with plan B, but Dr. D does not say this last part. They know. It needs to sink in, and Dr. D is there with and for them in this moment.

Projecting into the Future with Transplantation

Dr. D does not leave, he waits, and it is Mrs Spencer who takes the turn after a few seconds of silence. She asks a question relating to Ms Moose's book about her experience with Giant Cell Myocarditis and her family journey through heart transplantation. Somebody has told Mrs Spencer that it is best for the family but not for Mr Spencer to read the book.

466	Dr. D:	well I would uh
467		in this case as you feel
468		when (.) from this probably also
469		but probably also from another book that (.)
470		you should have talked about
471		this relational medicine book
472		that there's a certain role distribution um
473		that I feel us white coats make recommendations
474		and the boss makes decisions
475		then the boss happens to be the young man (.)
476		so IF you want to read that
477		there's no reason not to (.)
478	Wife:	because he's the boss
479	Dr. D:	yes (.) over *his* life
480		and his rule number one is
481		listen to my wife *((Dr. D gestures quotation marks for this utterance))*
482		which is in this case yours (3.0)
483	Wife:	so who is the boss then
484		ha[haha
485	Dr. D:	[that's a good question
		((Smiley voice))
486		see
487		that's the dialectics of couple relationships (.8)
488		now you figure that out (2.3)

Dr. D and Mrs Spencer joke. Mr Spencer is silent. And then, he asks about the symptoms after the heart transplantation surgery. He treads slowly. The long silences are interrupted neither by the physician nor by his wife.

494	Mr. Spencer:	with the heart transplant (3.8) (clears throat)
495		assuming that you get a pretty healthy heart (.8)
496		how (2.6) how quickly does (3.0)
497		like the lightheadedness
498		and the (.8) water retention
499		and the weakness
500		start to (.4) feel normal again (.6)
501		and the cough? (.6)
502		and (2.0) all the things associated with it
503		I mean (.) like (.)
504		would you wake up and
505		all of a sudden just realize (1.5)
506		there's obviously
507		they've cut into your chest (.)
508		but (.9) like (.6)

509		my wits are about me again
510		there's blood in my head I can
511	Dr. D:	mhmm
512	Mr Spencer:	is it (1.2) fairly quick o:r
513	Dr. D:	yes (1.1)
514		within days (2.2)

Yes, "within days" is the answer Dr. D gives to Mr Spencer's first question about AdHF symptoms after heart transplantation surgery. Two seconds pause, and then Dr. D continues.

515	Dr. D:	keep in mind
516		regardless of what kind of (.7)
517		donor organ you receive
518		it's always a healthy donor organ um
519		that is matched (.8) to you
520		in that you live decades with it
521		you know
522	Mr. Spencer:	mhm mhm

Dr. D responds to what he knows to be not only Mr Spencer's doubt about receiving a "healthy donor organ" but of many patients he had cared for (lines 516–518). "Then Dr. D continues with postoperative recovery, the waking up from the surgery, and the need to get extubated as soon as possible "to communicate um *meaning*fully (.)" to really *get out* of the intensive care unit **soon**" (lines omitted).

547	Mr. Spencer:	yeah I mean I don't know if I could
548		handle a tube down my throat any other way
549	Dr. D:	and that's why we are very interested
550		in having the tube out of your airways
551		very quickly after heart transplantation (1.4)
552		you know (.) often the attempt is
553		within the first uh twenty four hour period (3.3)
554		and uh the only thing by the way
555		to really prepare for that on your part is (.5)
556		and I'm looking for this (.6) device uh to
557		use your incentive spirometer
558		this little white blue plastic tool
559		where you do (.9) five-minutes-per-hour-
560		ten-hours-per-day
561		inha:ling exercise to pull the little ball
562		to the position that says
563		best (1.2) that expands your lungs
564	Mr. Spencer:	okay

Mr Spencer is so repelled by anything invading his body that even the idea of being intubated for surgery and waking up with a breathing tube can be a reason to avoid surgery altogether. Dr. D talks faster (lines 565–566; 568–569), possibly to prevent an interruption:

```
565    Dr. D:    a:nd uh is exactly the-kind-of-exercise-that-
566              you-need when you wake up
567              and then the (.5) team wants you to
568              have the tube-out-of-your-airways
569              and then you-cough-up-all-the stuff
570              you need to be awake for that
571              so: the best preparation is
572              to (.) practice this (.6) now
573              and uh incentive spirometer.
574              so it should be in the room
575              but if it's not (.) then the nurse can (.7)
576              and should bring this to you (.8) you know
577              it should be actually (.5) standing more here
```

Raia (2020) discusses how projecting a person into future possibilities after having grounded the person in a common existential past is crucial in caring for another. Projecting Mr Spencer into imagining the actions he can take on a path toward recovery is a big step into Mr Spencer's existential future. Dr. D looks for the incentive spirometer, but he cannot find it in the room and asks the nurse to bring one to make Mr Spencer start his exercise. Mr Spencer is now ready for Dr. D to leave. Dr. D leaves with the promise of being back:

```
612    Mr. Spencer:    okay (.9) thank you doctor (1.0)
613                    thank you very much
614    Dr. D:          (2.4) okay
615                    (.5) I'll be back
```

December 31

The nurse steps outside Mr Spencer's room and walks toward Dr. D. She is worried. Dr. D asks her to walk with him and the AdHF Fellow to the briefing with the primary GC team assembled at the nursing station; he wants to talk to the GC team before entering Mr Spencer's room.

Mr Spencer is not doing well this morning. He had nausea and vomited. CCU Nurse N thinks that it results from fluid overload and impaired oxygen delivery secondary to the progression of the disease. Mr Spencer's Systemic Vascular Resistance (SVR) is very high; this means that the blood pressure–lowering medications required a further increase (uptitration), as we learned from the discussion about titrating medication on the day before. Mr Spencer was crying this morning. "He was crying and felt he was in such a mess." CCU Nurse N tries to console him, reminding him that only 3 weeks ago, he was putting up the lights on the Christmas tree. What happened is such a traumatic event. He is expected to feel overwhelmed, "a mess," as Mr Spencer described his state. CCU Nurse N looks down, closes her eyes, and shakes her head while inhaling deeply; she is visibly moved by or maybe worried about Mr Spencer's situation. Mr Spencer, she continues, is also now very aware that the situation is not evolving in the direction he hoped for. Dr. D, with a somber tone, agrees, the situation is becoming urgent. They approach the nursing station discussing it. They need to coordinate with Dr. S, the assigned AdHF surgeon. The GC Attending calls Dr. S. The multidisciplinary team caring for Mr Spencer stands around the nursing station. Dr. S is not in the hospital but on speakerphone. Dr. D and the GC Attending believe that Mr Spencer's condition is spiraling downward. Yet, they do not want Dr. S to think that the situation requires his immediate presence for an emergency Biventricular Assist Device (BiVAD) implantation. So, after having updated Dr. S about Mr Spencer's current condition, they jokingly add "you can continue to do your shopping." "I am not shopping," laughs Dr. S, "yees yees" Dr. D and the GC Attending jokingly rebut, it is, after all, December 31, a time for celebration with family and friends with champagne and good food. "You can continue your shopping" communicates that while there is a transition toward an urgent situation, it is not an emergency.

Dr. D knocks at the door of Mr Spencer's CCU room.

1	Mr. Spencer:	hello:?
		(8.0)
2		how are you today
3	Dr. D:	I feel good (2.0)
4		having slept for six hours (1.8)
5		and um (1.7)
6		having had the pri*vileg*e of rounding ((smiley voice))
7		in the ho:spital this morning (2.0) ((smiley voice))
8		and before doing so
9		having to send out an email to our (0.7)
10		AD HOC committee? to (0.9) um
11		complete our listing process with you:? (1.0)
12		and so we prepa:red for (0.5) the scenarios

13		that uh (0.7) you know (0.4) could come up
14		and having talked to [HTx Coordinator]
15		our financial coordinator to prophylactically make all
16		the (0.4) clearance preparations
17		for the ventricular assist device
18		should-it-become neces*sary*, (1.0) you know (0.8)
19		and at the s*A*me time um hearing the team's view
20		[unudible]
21		so it's it's
22		living with this um interpretation of the course (0.5)
23		in a kind of (1.0) m*o*ment by m*o*ment basis
24		that's what I'm actually (0.7) in right now in my mind (2.0)
25	Mr. Spencer:	okay
		((*softly spoken*))
26	Dr. D:	and y*ou:*

Mr Spencer's first utterance is a question for Dr. D, how is Dr. D doing today? Mr Spencer's question is uttered with a somber tone and met by Dr. D's cheerful and smiley voice. As a researcher, who is studying their interactions, I am surprised. After the discussion at the nursing station about the accelerating urgency of Mr Spencer's heart failure condition, the nurse's description of his emotional state, and knowing Dr. D to be a very empathic and compassionate person, I had expected Dr. D to enter attuned to the situation, matching Mr Spencer's existential disappointment and fear for his life. But that is not what is happening. I worry that Mr Spencer will be taken aback by Dr. D's response; he could feel that the doctor does not care for his existential worries and be taken aback as I am.

"Having" (line 4), "having" (line 6), "having" (line 9); as it erupted, my worry subsides. I am taken into a rhythm of what's up next (lines 10–23). Dr. D is at ease in the situation describing the steps taken this morning as routine steps. He is very comfortable with them, I feel reassured, and it finally dawns on me that it is precisely what Dr. D is doing. He is reassuring Mr Spencer. "We have you." "We are here with you, and we know what we are doing." This time, contrary to what we have seen in the encounter on December 29 with the GC Fellow in training (Chapter 4), the message that Mr Spencer is in capable hands does not carry the loss of agency for Mr Spencer. It is a caring power voice guiding Mr Spencer to address the impending issue:

27	Mr. Spencer:	(1.4) um (1.0) it sounds to me: (1.3) like
28		urh urh ((*clears his thought*))

29		it's taking more and more stimulants
30		to keep this heart (0.7) **doing** what it needs to do
31		and so that's not the trend that we were looking for (0.8)
32		so I a**m** prepared for plan **B**? if that's what it takes (3.0)
33		and u::h (3.5)
34		that actually indicates kind of where the things might be so=
35	Dr. D:	=uhm-uhm

Mr Spencer responds to Dr. D's question (line 25) and addresses the issue of having to be prepared for plan B "if that is what it takes" (line 31). Mr Spencer remains silent even after Dr. D's continuer "uhm-uhm" inviting him to talk. What does Dr. D think?

36		(2.5)
37	Dr. D:	agree (0.9)
38		and you know how it was: you know
39		in the morning um meeting team meeting
40		and we're kind of continuously uhm (.) updating that
41		uhm (.) yeah I think it's important that these (.) ((sigh))
42		going and working through this
43		and while that's going on obviously
44		we continue the immunosuppressive uh therapy
45		um how have you been um at night
46		did you get some sleep

Dr. D treads carefully again (lines 36–40) and sighs; it is important to work through this, to accept plan B. After Dr. D's question about how Mr Spencer has slept, doctor and patient talk about the night. Mr Spencer reports what CCU Nurse N has already discussed with Dr. D; however, Dr. D neither interrupts nor says he already knows; he asks probing questions and listens to Mr Spencer's narrative:

47	Mr. Spencer:	so but still the ((clears throat))
48		the trend is tiring so (3.16)
49		I guess there's no predicting really (.5)
50		how long you could hold out this way (.8) right?
51	Dr. D:	that's right
52		it's very difficult to predict (1.2)
53		it's very difficult (1.0)
54		clearly um every one of **us** (.8) in the (.5) in the team
55		and uh from the discussions (.9) you know um (.6)
56		as we always do um (.5) in our decision making
57		has a s**EN**se (.8) you know which direction and
58		that's very much um (.6) concordant with what you

59	just described of your *sen*se (1.2) and that
60	that is often a very important uh information
61	although you can't quantitate that exactly (.6)
62	you know? (1.2)
63	but that's important (1.8)
64	and that means just (.6) getting pr*epa*:red (1.)
65	um that's all I think that is
66	actually ***necessary*** right now
67	because if you're (.5) as I said
68	scenario one scenario two or option-one-option-two
69	prepared for bo:th (1.1) and you see that
70	let's say from one-moment-to-the-next
71	the *LI*KElihoods of (.7) one option
72	going towards option one
73	option two are changing then you're prepared
74	so that's (.5) all one's need to do:: right now
75	but that's um where you feel the atmosphere (.7)
76	not allowing for just relaxing
77	leaning back and enjoying the ride (.6)
78	that's ***not*** the mindset
79	it's really (.5) pro*acti*vely getting prepared (.9)
80	you know

Mr Spencer returns to the question of how long his heart can be stable. Dr. D's response does not minimize the role that uncertainty plays in making sense of the complexity and ambiguity of health conditions in the process of decision-making for the team (lines 51–56) and Mr Spencer (lines 57–60). Within a dynamic situation, the comparison between the two plans is ongoing (line 69), as the doctors have just discussed at the nursing station. It is *necessary* (line 66) for all to be pre*pa*red (line 64); this includes Mr Spencer, not an object which the team soon will act upon but an agent "pro*acti*vely getting prepared" (line 79).

Dr. D explains in cogen that this "proactively getting prepared," based on the team's probabilistic reasoning through future scenarios, allows talking with Mr Spencer about the plans without forcing a decision on Mr Spencer's part. Indeed, Dr. D explains further that in his experience with Mr Spencer, the decision to accept transplantation can be embraced only as a possibility for Mr Spencer as he is sensing a potential change into a more urgent situation himself. Maintaining the uncertainty open in front of Mr Spencer has the effect of preventing rejection of the option. As Dr. D has spoken of the familiar and framed plan A and plan B as plan one and plan two,

Mr Spencer's wife asks for clarification, and Dr. D reassumes the two options with the resolved nomenclature. Mr Spencer continues:

```
81   Mr. Spencer:   I'm I'm mentally there already so (1.4)
                    ((clears throat))
82                  (2.4) I (1.0) need (.) I've said this a lot of times
83                  that I like to know what's going on
84                  I feel like everybody's kept me very informed (.9)
85                  and it HElps me cross this bridge (1.5)
86                  because I can (1.0) see what's going on myself so (4.2)
87                  so when's the next time you update the list?
```

Mr Spencer is mentally there. He agrees with the doctors as they kept him informed and at pace with the evolving situation. The team actions have helped Mr Spencer making an incredible step that, as he had expressed (segment 3.1 and 3.3, Chapter 3), meant crossing the existential bridge of accepting plan B he thought he could not accept. Mr Spencer asks a question about the timing of the heart transplant listing decision "when's the next time you update the list?" (line 87). Not returning back to immunosuppressive medications or his pacemaker (as seen on December 30), but taking a step toward Plan B.

```
88   Dr. D:   oh that's uh right now in the process
89            uh as I said I sent the communication
90            to the (.7) team members uh
91            and uh it's now (1.1) you know
92            in lieu of what we usually do
93            when we meet every Friday morning at seven o'clock
94            (.9) all thirty persons (1.2) uh because it's you know
95            between two Friday meetings and (.6) in addition
96            between the years u::h we have the mechanism
97            the ad hoc mechanism works by email (1.9) you know
98            the responses are coming back (2.)
```

Dr. D continues by explaining the nature of multidisciplinary teamwork during the evaluation and recommendation-making process. The team includes 75 professionals, AdHF cardiologists, surgeons, nurses, transplant coordinators, social workers, psychiatrists, case coordinators, quality officers, immunologists, infection disease physicians, palliation team members, and pharmacists. Each Friday, they are invited, as a selection committee, to discuss each case in detail and make decisions regarding the therapeutic options. Not all need to attend each meeting. Usually, 30 to 40 professionals attend. There are two situations in which the process has exceptions: one occurs when the urgency of the patient's condition cannot wait until the meeting takes place on the following Friday. The other occurs when the meeting is not taking place because of a holiday. In Mr Spencer's case, both conditions apply. In these cases, an email-based ad hoc mechanism is initiated by the AdHF Attending on record. The ad hoc is a formal decision-making mechanism involving all the relevant healthcare decision-makers — AdHF attending cardiologist and surgeon assigned to the patient, the surgical and medical directors of the transplant program, infection disease specialist, psychiatrist, nurse specialists, social worker, and pharmacist. Mr Spencer and Dr. D talk (lines omitted) about the listing, the role of the infection disease Attending in monitoring the possible risk factors, and the contraindications due to Mr Spencer's high dose of immunosuppressant therapy for his Giant Cell Myocarditis that makes his medication regime similar to the treatment after transplantation.

Then, Dr. D reins in the "scenario planning" (line 254) for the possibility of a bridge to transplantation via mechanical assist device(s):

252	Dr. D:	mhmm (2.8) yeah (2.8)
253		to um (1.0) come back to the whole
254		(1.5) scenario planning (.8)
255		then if assist heart pump (.)
256		there are different types (2.4)
257		and we talked about this already
258		and um (1.6) uh (1.8) Dr. S (.5)
259		one of the heart surgeon colleagues um
260		is also looking at that right now you know um
261		the main uh (1.1) distinction between these pumps
262		is really um is this only requiring
263		support for the left side of the heart
264		which is the *left* (.7) ventricle (1.5) uh
265		or for left and right ventricle (1.1)
266		and um (1.9) maybe there's some chance that it
267		will require for the left and right ventricle (1.4)
268		and um (1.4) there are different ways of uh (1.1)
269		uh doing that

Dr. D refers to a previous conversation (line 257) at the beginning of their relationship. Dr. D discusses (lines omitted) the four main options as part of the bridge to transplantation in plan B. He starts from the three options that Dr. D knows Mr Spencer does not want: the combination of HeartMate2, a left ventricular pump implanted inside the body that connects to the portable computer and batteries through a driveline out of the belly wall, and a Centrimag device, to support the right ventricle, whose pump is outside the body making the blood circulation visible to the patient designed for short-term use within the hospital. Using this combination, however, Mr Spencer cannot go home to recover. The second option is a Paracorporeal Ventricular Assist Device (PVAD) BiVAD with both left and right device's pumps outside the body but allowing Mr Spencer to go home to recover and wait for transplantation. Mr Spencer does not like to see his blood recycled through the pumps hanging outside his body. The third is the total artificial heart.

294	Dr. D:	and the third one would be the total artificial heart
295		which uh is the most (.6) let's say (.7)
296		I don't want to say aggressive or radical one
297		but it is a replacement device
298		it's not an assist heart pump (1.1)
299		and uh we have discussed that already
300		and I have your (1.1) good sense of your
301		intuitive first response to that (2.2)
302		and so that's uh (.) that's the
303		those scenarios you know (2.0)
304	Mr. Spencer:	yeah the left assist or even a left and right assist
305	Dr. D:	mhmm
306	Mr. Spencer:	I'm willing to do but the artificial heart or
307		an external heart pump
308		or anything like that I don't (2.2) ((clears throat)) (2.0)

Mr Spencer reiterates his choices (line 306–308): no external heart pump or artificial heart. One other available option exists: a HeartWare device for both ventricles, the HeartWare pumps are implantable and Mr Spencer can go home. Dr. D left this option as the last of the four options, the one that, from what he has been learning from Mr Spencer, could be the preferable choice (line omitted). Is it a coincidence? In Chapter 4, we discussed how Dr. D uses caring power to make certain possibilities acceptable. We asked Dr. D in cogen about this passage. His first reaction was a surprised, joyfully, and mischievous laughter. It left no doubt with us: he had constructed the list of the four options purposely based on his knowledge of Mr Spencer's way of life, view of the world, and concerns with futility in high-tech medicine. Indeed, Mr Spencer had indicated that to keep his heart, he would have considered accepting to live a life attached to a mechanical device. His second desire was to go home as soon as possible, and the third, to avoid seeing his blood circulating in the pumps. It is interesting to point out that Dr. D presents the options from bad (remaining in the hospital and visible blood circulating in the pumps) to worse (artificial heart, substituting Mr Spencer's heart completely with a machine). Within this frame, accepting the fourth option feels almost like a relief. Soft power or caring power? For Dr. D, the desired outcome is not to gain recognition of his or the team's cultural values (soft power). Dr. D and the team need to support Mr Spencer "crossing this bridge" with the BiVAD that, in Dr. D's understanding of Mr Spencer's lifeworld, is more conducive to his best and safest recovery. Dr. D's goal translates into taking Mr Spencer through progressively less attractive perspectives before presenting what he considers the best option for Mr Spencer.

Then, Mr Spencer asks the same question he asked the day before about waking up from surgery intubated. However, this time, the question is related to the bridge to transplantation. Together again, Dr. D and Mr Spencer imagine the action Mr Spencer can take toward the recovery as an essential step into Mr Spencer's existential future. Dr. D this time uses the incentive spirometer, which, in the meantime, has been brought into Mr Spencer's room. Together they work through the exercise and the explanation of its value and effectiveness.

447	Mr. Spencer:	I think (1.5) for me I'm (1.1) I'm up for it
448		but I'd just be honest
449		being intubated and conscious (1.1) is a (1.4)
450		more scary than dying
451		not really ((clears throat))
452		we are (1.1) um (1.5) christian people and
453		I have (.7) a strong faith of (1.8)
454		when this life is over
455		and if this is (.) the number of my days
456		that God had for me (.6)
457		I don't fear that
458		I'd like to still be a husband and a father
459		for a good long time ((clears throat))
460		but uh (1.9) intubation is
461		I've already laid here
462		through a lot of things but (.8)
463		being conscious with a tube down my throat
464		and (1.1) it's a little scary (1.) but=
465	Dr. D:	=agree

466	Mr. Spencer:	uh I'm sure I'm sure there's (.9)
467		sedatives and stuff
468		still involved after consciousness
469	Dr. D:	yes (2.1) I agree (2.4)
470		that's why it's the uh goal
471		that (.5) once you wake up
472		that this the tube is out
473		as soon as possible (1.2) you know
474		and that's why the preparation
475		for that moment is so important
476		and that is homework
477		you can do right now
478		it's among the most important things (.7)
479		in addition to (.6) um
480		doing kind of physical exercises (1.1)
481		and uh talking through with everybody (.)
482		that's the best preparation for
483		whatever uh exactly is coming up (1.1)
484		you know (3.)
485	Mr. Spencer:	okay

Mr Spencer shares with his doctor the fear of waking up having a tube down his throat. It goes so much against his sense of being that he finds it scarier than death. Dr. D agrees (line 469). He agrees not on finding it so scary himself, but on the understanding that something can be perceived as a threat to one's own being and immediately projects Mr Spencer on things he can do, things that move the image of being intubated and powerless, into images of actions reinforcing Mr Spencer's sense of agency and participation as an active subject in the situation. "Okay," concludes Mr Spencer.

"I will be back," Dr. D will see him tomorrow.

CHAPTER 6
INCREASING URGENCY

On January 1, Mr Spencer's condition is deteriorating fast. Only 3 days ago, heart transplantation was just a possible scenario that the team and Mr Spencer were hoping to avoid. Then it became a reality. Yesterday, with the sudden deterioration of Mr Spencer's condition, the dreaded option of a bridge to transplantation with the implantation of machines (Ventricular Assist Devices [VADs]) that everybody thought was avoidable became the new reality. As Dr. D and Mr Spencer discussed 3 days ago and again yesterday, before the deterioration of Mr Spencer's condition, this extra next step will require Mr Spencer to undergo VAD implantation surgery.

While recovering from it, Mr Spencer will be temporarily delisted from the active heart transplantation list and listed as United Network for Organ Sharing (UNOS) Status 7–Temporarily not Transplantable. Being UNOS Status 7 often provokes considerable anxiety in patients who fear that their condition could worsen and deteriorate and they would die before heart transplantation. The emotional connection that patients establish thinking about "their" heart and not "a" generic heart becoming available also provokes anxiety not to be able to receive 'their' heart because they are still on UNOS 7 status (Raia & Deng, 2015b). After recovering from machine implantation, Mr Spencer will possibly be discharged from the hospital and reactivated for the active heart transplantation list. Then, the active waiting period for a heart offer starts ... a liminal space, a place of transition. Patients and their families report that they are caught between hope for an offer of a donor heart, guilt knowing that the heart offer requires someone else's death, another family's tragedy, and ongoing concern about their own current, fragile status.

Dr. D knows all this. He had been in touch over the phone with Dr. S, the Advanced Heart Failure (AdHF) surgeon, about the evolving situation. They both agreed to proceed with mechanical circulatory support as a bridge to heart transplantation to support both left and right ventricles. Four mechanical device options are suitable: a Paracorporeal Biventricular Assist Device (PVAD-BiVAD), Left Ventricular Assist Device (LVAD) Heart-ware/Right Ventricular Assist Device (RVAD) Centrimag combination, a Total Artificial Heart (TAH), or the HeartWare BiVAD (HVAD-BiVAD). Dr. D and Mr Spencer talked about them yesterday, today, and they will discuss them again with Dr. S and Mr Spencer's family.

Dr. D is on his CCU rounds with the trainee, the AdHF Fellow, and preparing to enter Mr Spencer's room. He hears the steady voice of Dr. S, the AdHF surgeon, talking to Mr Spencer.

1	Dr. S:	When you've reached this point
2		you have a few options a:nd

Mr Spencer lies in the hospital bed. The room feels crowded by the number of people, the monitors, and infusion lines gathered around Mr Spencer. (Fig. 6.1).

The number of lines and tubes reaching Mr Spencer's bed and disappearing under his sheet crowding around him seem to have increased. He is now receiving numerous continuous infusions, some of them added today (Fig. 6.2).

Dr. D's and the AdHF Fellow's entry does not interrupt the conversation between Dr. S and Mr Spencer. Dr. S has come to introduce himself and meet his new patient, Mr Spencer. Dr. S needs to discuss with Mr Spencer the different options to reach a decision and then consent Mr Spencer. It will be Dr. S who will coordinate and conduct Mr Spencer's heart surgeries: the machine implantation (VAD) first and the heart transplantation later.

As Dr. S discusses in cogen session, it is essential for him to meet Mr Spencer before the surgery:

Dr. S: "my personal philosophy is that ... opening somebody up ... there's not many levels of intimacy that go beyond a surgeon-patient relationship, so I always try to spend some time communicating because if you don't do that, then I just don't see how that relationship can be effectual and long term. You know, the caricature is that we cut [...] But I just think of myself a lot

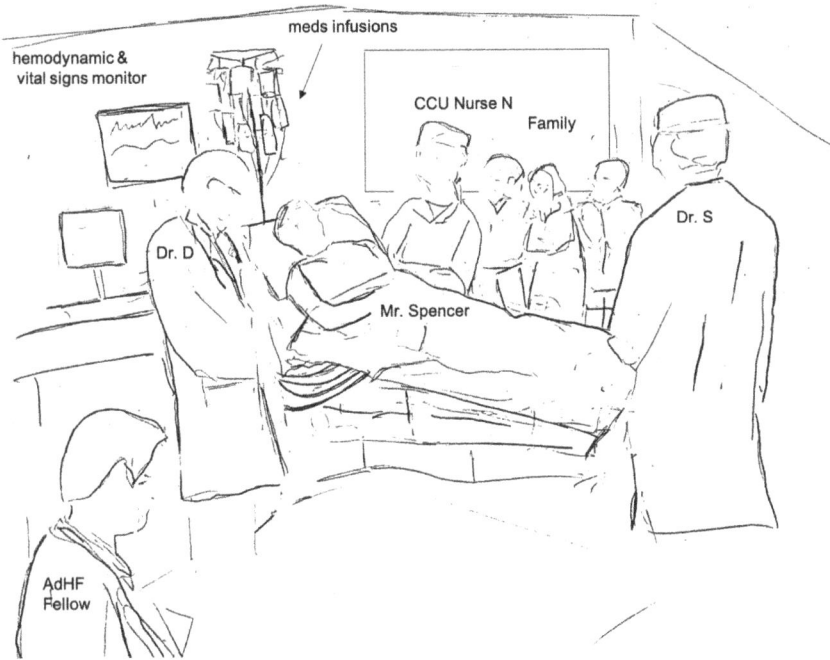

Figure 6.1: Mr Spencer's CCU hospital room. The recorder is on the shelf between Dr. D and Mr Spencer. Dr. S, at the foot of the bed, faces Mr Spencer. CCU Nurse N is on Mr Spencer's left side. Behind her stand Mr Spencer's wife and brother, behind them, his father. The AdHF Fellow, who has come in with Dr. D, remains near the door. Dr. D walks toward Mr Spencer. He puts his notes on the cart holding the computer at the right side of the bed and joins the inner circle of healthcare professionals primarily responsible for Mr Spencer's care plan, Dr. S and CCU Nurse N, around the bed.

more . . . multi-dimensional. As a surgeon, you do carry some ability to offer emotional and psychological consolation. So I think if that's something that I can do, then I should do it. [. . .] For example, I feel that it is very important that I talk to the patient before they're put to sleep. They need to see my face before they are put to sleep. I adhere to this, almost without exception; although not all surgeons feel it is important. Many times when surgeons enter the OR [Operating Room], the patient is already under anesthesia. But I think it's very important that I hold their hand, tell them there are doing fine, ask if they have questions. And that's the same here. How you talk

Medications:
Scheduled Meds:

- acyclovir   400 mg Intravenous   Q24H
- amiodarone bolus   150 mg Intravenous   Once
- amiodarone   400 mg Oral   BID
- cotrimoxazole DS   1 tablet Oral   Once per day on Mon Wed Fri
- diphenhydramine IVPB   50 mg   Intravenous   Once
- docusate   100 mg Oral   BID
- doxycycline   100 mg Intravenous   Q12H
- fluconazole IV   200 mg Intravenous   Q24H
- heparin 5,000 Units   Subcutaneous   BID
- lidocaine   1 mg/kg (Dosing Weight) Intravenous   Once
- lidocaine
- [START ON *((in two days))* date removed] methylprednisolone IV   16 mg   Intravenous   Once
- [START ON *((following day))* date removed] methylprednisolone IV 24 mg   Intravenous   Once
- mycophenolate   1,000 mg   Intravenous   BID
- pantoprazole   40 mg   IV Push Q24H
- pneumococcal polyvalent vaccine 0.5 mL Intramuscular   Once
- polyethylene glycol   17 g   Oral   Daily
- tacrolimus   0.5 mg Oral   BID

Continuous Infusions:

- amiodarone 600 mg/ 100 mL drip (Central) 0.5 mg/min (01/01/)
- anticoagulant citrate dextrose (ACD-A)
- anticoagulant citrate dextrose (ACD-A)
- anticoagulant citrate dextrose (ACD-A)
- lidocaine   0.5 mg/min (01/01/)
- milrinone   0.2 mcg/kg/min (01/01/)
- nitroprusside drip 100 mg/250 mL (400 mcg/mL)   1.385 mcg/kg/min (01/01/1)
- norepinephrine drip   Stopped (12/21/)
- sodium chloride 10 mL/hr (12/28/)

PRN Meds:.benzonatate, bisacodyl, bupivacaine-epinephrine PF, insulin aspart **AND** dextrose, guaifenesin, non formulary, ondansetron, promethazine-codeine, simethicone, sodium chloride

Figure 6.2: Excerpt from the AdHF daily note written by the AdHF Fellow and co-signed by the AdHF Attending cardiologist: Mr Spencer's current list of medications.

to the patient in the preoperative phase, which includes getting informed consent *(such as the situation right here in Mr. Spencer's room)*, it's a relationship-building exercise. I think if you miss that opportunity, you do your practice a real true disservice because you can offer so much more to a patient other than the ability to cut and sew ..."

Meeting the Surgeon

In Mr Spencer's CCU room, Dr. S continues to discuss the current situation and the options. With Mr Spencer and his family, we have got to know them as plan A and plan B. However, this time, it is Dr. S, an AdHF surgeon, who discusses them. It is common for an AdHF surgeon like Dr. S to meet a new patient in urgency, if not emergency, situations like this. Today, Dr. S needs to introduce himself to Mr Spencer and his family, establish a trustful relationship with them while discussing the options that he, as a surgeon, considers the best. Dr. S needs to discuss all the possibilities, even if he knows that Mr Spencer and his family had discussed them with other team members. It is with Dr. S's surgical perspective that the journey needs to be shared. Mr Spencer and his family need to understand how other members of the team approach and discuss the various options as healthcare professionals who care for them.

3	Dr. S:	one of them i:s
4		to go straight to transplant u:hh
5		but th:e problem with that option (.)
6		is that (.) we don't h:ave
7		ready access to organs and
8		we are not sure
9		what the time frame will be
10		in most cases it takes weeks if (.) not (.) months

Heart transplantation. When? Nobody knows when. A heart compatible with Mr Spencer's blood type, immune system, and body size will need to become available. Nobody can predict when. A person's death, donating his or her heart, is a necessary condition for heart transplantation to be possible. Mr Spencer knows it. His family knows it. There is no need to talk about it in these terms. This knowledge hovers in the room and will always be a presence for Mr Spencer and his family as it is for other heart transplantation patients and their families (O. Mauthner *et al.*, 2012; Shildrick, 2012, 2015).

The hesitation (u:hh, line 4) and the micropauses (line 5, 6, and 10) are suggestive of the "delicate" nature of this conversation (Silverman & Peräkylä, 1990). Dr. S's steady way of talking is punctuated by the elongation of vowels of some words, similar to what Beach (2014) shows in oncology medical encounters. This elongation creates a brief suspension before the following words are uttered, marking both the importance and the delicacy of what is spoken afterward (underlined here): "i:s to go straight to transplant" (lines 3–4); "th:e problem with that option" (line 5); and "don't h:ave ready access to organs" (lines 6–7). The micropauses (.) on lines 5, 6, and 10, have a similar effect.

11	Dr. S:	but there is no way to predict (.)
12		if you will be able to **physi**cally be o**ka**y
13		while we're waiting for that heart (.) so
14		I'm sure you have heard
15		about the devices we have used (.)
16		to get people to that point we call that
17		bridge to transplant
18		we bridge people to transplant
19		with devices that
20		allow you to feel better
21		allow you to kinda of recover
22		your body to recover
23		to get strong again and then
24		going to transplant
25		as healthy as you possibly can **b:e**
26		because your body
27		is receiving the blood flow it needs
28		to work effectively
29		which in this current case
30		it's not

In Dr. S' talk, which is otherwise steady, the short micropauses (.) on lines 11, 13, and 15 give the feeling of a talk treading carefully through the VADs implantation option. This new reality is inexorably sinking into Mr Spencer's life. Short pauses disappear after line 15. Now, in each sentence, a word is repeated as if making it familiar. In each sentence, a new aspect is added for Mr Spencer to make sense of the benefit derived from the implantation of machines: for example, the "*bridge* to *transplant*" on line 17 becomes "we *bridge* people to *transplant*" on line 18 and then "going to *transplant* as healthy as you possibly can **b:e**" on line 24; on lines 20 to 21, devices "that *allow* you to feel better" "*allow* you to kinda of *recover*" and "your body to *recover* and to get strong again" (lines 22–23). As we saw done by Dr. D in Chapter 3, now is Dr. S creating a rhythm to take Mr Spencer into the new unknown path. And then Dr. S concludes (line 29): "which [your body] in this current case it's not," preparing for a new step, a more urgent one.

On razor's edge

31	Dr. S:	Although I ***MUST*** SAY
32		your numbers look okay you're
33		((inaudible))
34		uuhh but i do think you're
35		on uh razor's edge
36		you are on a margin right now and
37		any little wind can blow you
38		over to the opposite thin line
39		you are walking on right now
40		and then
41		we can end worse off
42		than we are now
43		you can end up back on the ecmo
44		either on ecmo or some other device
45		that's actually a step back

URGENCY OF THE SITUATION

The situation is urgent. Currently, Mr Spencer is stable; however, the health practitioners monitor the situation very closely, concerned for the arrhythmias to reappear or another "Code Blue." If that happens, the team needs to escalate from an urgent situation to an emergency. One team member will immediately initiate Cardiopulmonary Resuscitation (CPR), a hard and fast manual rhythmic cardio-compression with no interruptions to "maximize the number of compressions delivered per minute" (ECC Task Forces of the American Heart Association, 2005). One member will expose and prepare Mr Spencer's chest for electric shocks; another will rush in the crash-cart from the CCU hallway to use the Automatic External Defibrillator (AED): Clear! All will raise their hands to show no contact with Mr Spencer's body. CPR stops. All clear. The AED will electrically shock Mr Spencer's heart into resuming its normal rhythm; CPR resumes immediately afterwards. The guidelines (American Heart Association, 2005) are clear, 30 compressions before a second shock. Clear!

If Mr Spencer's heart does not resume its regular beating while the cardio-compression continues, the team will "prepare for ECMO." ECMO stands for Extra-Corporeal Membrane Oxygenator (Rao *et al.*, 2018). It is an artificial heart and lung machine requiring the insertion of two cannulae for infusion and drainage (Napp *et al.*, 2016). The venous cannula, usually inserted from the groin in the femoral vein, takes venous blood from the low blood pressure vessel, the vein, into the ECMO. In the ECMO, two things happen: (1) carbon dioxide is eliminated, and oxygen is added (oxygenation); this is the lung function of the ECMO (also called gas exchange function); (2) the oxygenated blood is pumped with high pressure into the body via the arterial cannula, usually inserted in the groin artery. Based on the functionality of this circuit, the ECMO was initially called the heart-lung machine (Punjabi & Taylor, 2013). After calling the ECMO team, Mr Spencer would need to be prepared for intubation. Under emergency conditions, it is challenging to "find access to the blood vessels" to insert the cannula into the vein and artery: the lack of pulse from the absent heartbeats pumping blood from and into the vessels precludes an unambiguous localization of the blood vessels. For example, the pulsating flow in the artery, utilized to locate the vessel's position, cannot be used. There is no time to locate it with elective ultrasound examination but only with an orienting emergency examination while the manual cardio-compression generates the pulse. So, while a member of the team continues the rhythmic cardio-compression and another team member, at the head of the bed, manually operates the ventilator, the surgeon would carefully insert the cannulae from the groin. In emergencies, the chance of correct and efficient cannulation of the vessels is reduced compared to nonemergency situations with possible severe complications, including perforation of the blood vessels and bleeding, arterial dissection, and distal ischemia (Makdisi & Wang, 2015). While the team would try to restore the Return of Spontaneous Circulation (ROSC), Mr Spencer could suffer brain damage and other forms of organ failure from which recovery can be difficult or impossible. While on ECMO, a substantial risk of other adverse events like bleeding, vascular complications, thromboembolic events, and infection exists (Makdisi & Wang, 2015). As a researcher, having learned all this, having seen it in action and described previously (Raia & Deng, 2015b), I (FR) can almost hear the brain gears of the healthcare providers in the room working through the possibility of having to call a Code Blue.

The situation is urgent.

What Dr. S "MUST say" (line 31) is that Mr Spencer's "numbers look okay." Currently, the situation looks stable. However, Dr. S. introduces the sense of urgency by bracketing what he "must say" into a contrasting opening "although" and a contrasting closing with "I do think you are on razor's edge." In doing so, the surgeon's talk expresses the instability and the urgency of the situation. The careful treading of his talk changes into a metaphor (lines 34–40). It evokes the image of someone driving on a rainy day on a slippery slope on the highway at 100 mph, feeling that everything is "okay," not perceiving the opening of the abyss right in front of him: an illusion of stability in a situation characterized by a high hazard probability. Yet, the frantic pace of an emergency ECMO implantation the team wishes to avoid does not transpire from Dr. S's tone of voice, remarkably low key for an observer.

46	Mr. Spencer:	What's ecmo	Mr. Spencer's QUESTION about ECMO
47	Dr. S:	ECMO is just uh	
48		It's just an artificial heart and lung machine	
49		that runs out here but	
50		it goes through long long tubing and	Dr. S' EXPLANATION
51		it's a very temporary fix	
52		it's not it's not anything that	
53		that we can run for a *long* period of time	
54	Mr. Spencer:	You *((inaudible))* do that	
55	Dr. S:	yes so	
56		we would prefer not have to do that	
57		but uh	
58		we do think that the VA:D is in your future	

The introduction of ECMO into the conversation is taken up by Mr Spencer's question (line 46). Dr. S describes it as an artificial heart and lung machine that temporarily can support Mr Spencer's heart and lung function. The "temporary fix" (line 51) is for several hours to a few days before complications start arising. It is, after all, another machine, a short-term bridge to a long-term bridge to heart transplantation. As Dr. S voices, the team sees Mr Spencer preferably directly with a VAD in his future (line 58). i.e., only one bridge rather than a bridge to a bridge to transplantation. The *dreaded* VAD implantation is transformed into a *good* single step bridge to transplantation. The optimistic projection, also recognized in communication in other clinical settings (Beach, 2009, 2014; Holt, 1993; Maynard, 2003), is performed here by enlisting the entire medical team seeing Mr Spencer with a VAD: "we do think that the VA:D is in your future." An optimistic future scenario after the pessimistic possible "setback" (line 45) with another code blue and ECMO: the VAD, a single-step bridge to heart transplantation. The step of living on the VAD before undergoing heart transplantation, first a remote, then a closer and dreaded possibility 3 days ago, accepted yesterday, is a certainty now.

The VAD is in your future

59	Mr. Spencer:	Left and right or left ⟶	Mr. Spencer's QUESTION on type of VADs
60	Dr. S:	so that's an interesting question	
61		that's a little bit of a judgement call	
62		S:o typically	
63		if somebody has your disease (.6) the the uh	
64		the myocarditis affects	
65		both ventricles indiscriminately	
66		they affect both s:o	
67		there is no reason to suspect that	Dr. S' EXPLANATION: Reasoning in a General case
68		your right side will work well and	
69		your left side will not	
70		it's just kinda	
71		it just affects the entire heart	
72		both sides so the textbook answer will say	
73		right-and-left particularly	
74		if someone is having arrhythmias because	
75		if you only have half of the heart supported	
76		if you go into v-tach situations	
77		you won't necessarily be protected by the devices	

The conversation continues with Mr Spencer introducing a question about the need for two machines, the right and left VADs, or the need for only the left VAD: "left and right or left" (lines 59). The others present in the room are listening.

Dr. S appreciates (line 60) Mr Spencer's question about what type of VAD he would need, given the particularity of the Giant Cell Myocarditis disease affecting both heart ventricles indiscriminately (lines 65–66). He refers to the different options of machine implantation (lines 62–77). The explanations of the surgeon are detailed. As he reflected in a cogen session, "every patient is different. Some patients say: 'doctor, do what you gotta do.' They would not want to have the conversation I am having with Mr Spencer. Mr Spencer was much more involved, even as sick as he was, and wanted the nuances of everything explained. You have to gauge the patient too, because, to some patients, I do a disservice if I get too detail-oriented. It just burns them. Peace of mind is essential."

Dr. S unfolds his reasoning by starting from a more general description of what "typically" (line 62) happens and the possible textbook (line 72) solutions relating to Mr Spencer's case of having ventricular tachyarrhythmias (v-tach, line 76). A big fear for Mr Spencer is whether he would still suffer from them after the machine implantation (line 78).

78	Mr. Spencer:	with the device can i still go into v-tach	Mr Spencer's QUESTION about V-tach on VAD
79	Dr. S:	If you can go into v-tach	
80		If you have *both* ventricles supported?	
81		it doesn't matter because your heart just	
82		at that point becomes a re*ce*ptacle for blood	
83		the devices are actually doing all the pumping	
84		see you can be in *v-fib*	
85		which is even worse	
86		the heart doesn't even do anything	Dr S' EXPLANATION
87		and your your body may not even know it	
88		because it's just the blood	
89		is still being pumped by the machines uhh	
90		obviously biventricular support	
91		is a bigger operation	
92		it has-carries a few more risks uhh	
93		but in certain cases in my opinion	
94		I have put in both assortments	
95		I think it's it's the more conservative	
96		and therefore safer option for some people umm	

After responding to Mr Spencer's question (line 78), Dr. S resumes his talk, reasoning for preferring BiVAD implantation (line 90). There are higher risks in the implantation (line 92) and different benefits compared to left ventricular support implantation (lines 90–92). Dr. S bridges the conversation about choosing the type of VADs in response to Mr Spencer's question (line 59) by explicitly referring to what he said before ("as I told you," line 101) and repeating similar wording ("textbook answer," line 102).

97		with that being said your	
98		when you look at now	Dr. S
99		if you individualize the care to you	Resumes reasoning
100		as uhm a *patie*nt	on VADs types in
101		I just told you	Mr Spencer's
102		what the textbook global answer is	specific case
103		for giant cell myocarditis but	
104		if I look at you *dire*ctly	
105		you have a few specifics where (0.6)	
106		there ma:y be some possibilities	
107		that (0.5) a left sided only situation might (0.4)	
108		work [uh it does in my opinion	
109	Mr Spencer:	[hmm	
110	Dr S:	carry higher theoretical risks	
111		but you do have a few things	
112		that I can see that (0.5) it might be feasible	
113		so that's where I would like to	
114		kinda take a look in the operating room and	
115		see how you do	
116		be prepared for biventricular support (0.5)	
117		but also consider (0.7)	
118		if you are one of the subgroups	
119		that may do well with just the left side	
120		only because there are benefits of keeping it	
121		just to the left side (0.6) I would consider that	

There are individually tailored possible solutions Dr. S sees for Mr Spencer. Dr. S's utterances again become interspersed with short pauses as if Dr. S were exploring the possibilities while talking to Mr Spencer, reasoning with him.

The "weekend effect"

122	Mr. Spencer:	You would be the surgeon (1.9)
123		(1.9)
124		and uhh (0.6)
125		it's New Year's day (3.6)
126		and I mean I wouldn't assume
127		you've got your best team here

Mr Spencer is worried. He is in a teaching hospital, and he is afraid that the healthcare professionals on call during the holidays, on New Year's Day (line 125), are not the best experts.

The CCU Nurse N recalls in cogen:

> [...] he would ask me every day, 'So what days are you off, are you are you working on the holidays?' You know, I think he felt generally that not everybody's gonna be around for the holidays, and I said 'we all have to work the holidays, and, you know, the doctors are the same.' He was always very concerned about who was going to be his team and who was going to be around, so we tried to keep continuity of care with him because of this incredible fear that he was not going to get the best attention because of the holidays.

Mr Spencer's concerns reflect the widespread knowledge of an increased risk of adverse outcomes for patients admitted to hospitals during holidays and weekends in different parts of the western world (Bell & Redelmeier, 2001; Dube *et al.*, 2014; Hedley *et al.*, 2019). Television networks, as well as popular science journals (e.g., Chodosh, 2018; CNN, 2018), report that holiday seasons "can be deadly for hospital patients." A growing body of research examines what has become known as the weekend effect for safety, policy implications, and financial implications of staffing. The question of the weekend effect points to the variability of the density of staffing and delivery of services (e.g., availability of lab draws, diagnostic imaging facilities, etc.). Although research shows no "weekend effect" mortality observed for cardiac transplantation surgeries (Chand *et al.*, 2019; Salimbangon *et al.*, 2019), Mr Spencer's question also shows distrust toward the level of expertise of the medical personnel. How does the hierarchical world of medicine regulate who is on call during the holidays?

In interactional dynamics, participants display sensitivity toward potentially embarrassing matters and mark topics as delicate by using a variety of interactional phenomena to mitigate the embarrassment (e.g., Heath, 1988; Maynard, 1991; Silverman, 1997). However, while Mr Spencer uses modal auxiliary verbs such as "would" and "wouldn't assume" (van Nijnatten & Suoninen, 2013) and pauses marking the topic as sensitive (Linell & Bredmar, 1996), differently to what has been observed in other work in medical encounters (Weijts *et al.*, 1993), he constructs a very direct question. He uses personal pronouns ("you") and does not mitigate the effect of his question.

We listened to this encounter in various contexts, in classes, during data sessions with linguist anthropologists, education researchers, and with doctors in training (residents and fellows). When we arrived at this passage, we recorded similar responses: widening eyes and raising eyebrows with a simultaneous exclamation of u:::hhh, o::::hhhh. When prompted to elaborate, the participants' responses fell into three not exclusive categories of explanations: (1) understanding Mr Spencer's fear, (2) surprise for his candor, and (3) expecting Dr. S to be offended by the suggestion that he and his team were not "the best team here" (line 127).

128	Dr. S:	(1.3)
129		We:ll there's a call team and
130		the call team is comprised of people I work
131		I work during regular hours but
132		they're not a special team
133		it's the same people they just
134		who just happens to be on call on new year's uhm
135		It's just so you're right there's not
136		but you know optimally
137		I would not like to go at two in the morning
138		just because people aren't as fresh then
139		as they are in the morning but
140		if you can *wait until* a certain time
141		there is some theoretical benefit there
142		but (.) we do these operations
143		because they tend to be some type of emergency
144		we do them at all *times* at days
145		during the night
146		as well as weekends

The disagreement with Mr Spencer's statement is evident by Dr. S's delayed response with an initial pause (line 128) followed by "we:ll" (Ogden, 2006;

Pomerantz, 1984) after Mr Spencer's question. However, here the situation is more complicated as the surgeon discusses in cogen session:

> Patients don't have a personal agenda. They just have a legitimate concern, and [. . .] you have to come back with an answer that is true, and that also acknowledges the concerns of the patient. I also put that question in the category "How old are you?" They look at you, and they see no gray hair or anything. Sometimes, interesting, you know, you get questions like that.
> FR: In the sense, they think you don't have enough experience?
> Dr. S: Yes. Another example is when they ask 'so I hear you have in this teaching hospital residents that practice here. Will a resident practice on me? And so what do I say? I cannot say no. Residents do not do transplants specifically but do other things. So I'll say: yes, it is true, this is a teaching hospital. Yes, it's true; we are indeed charged with training the next generation of surgeons, as I am myself. I was trained and now have trained many people. You can have my assurance, though, because I am the surgeon of record, that nothing is done without my direct visualization, observation, and approval. [..] Sometimes, my vantage point [in the OR] means that I have the best access and be the most effective. Sometimes it's the person across from me who has the best advantage, and that person is doing it. I will watch it and make sure it's the same stitch that I would have thrown. I will be there for all key portions of the operation. The resident is in no way allowed to practice alone. You have my word that if the situation exceeds the abilities of that resident, I take over. So that's an example. You must be truthful, and you cannot be dismissive or circumvent these questions because then you will lose the trust of the patient.

Dr. S does not contradict Mr Spencer. Mr Spencer is right ("you're right there's not," line 135); people are not fresh at 2 o'clock in the morning (I would not like to go at 2 in the morning, line 137). Dr. S takes what is right in Mr Spencer's understanding and reframes it for him; the surgeon operates a transformation from "not the best team "into "they are not a special team." The mark of a delicate situation is given by the use of "would" and "wouldn't" similar to what Mr Spencer had done, and by Dr. S, who is part of "the call team" distancing himself from it by using the indirect utterances: "a" call team (lines 129–130) and the pronoun "they" (lines 133 and 140).

147	Mr. Spencer:	And by now are you thinking today
148	Dr. S:	well there are a few logistical hurdles
149		that we still have to clear and then
150		there's one thing I would like to talk to you
151		in terms of the devices so

The conversation between Mr Spencer and Dr. S continues while in the background Dr. D, CCU Nurse N, and the AdHF Fellow talk.

Dr. S resumes the discussion initiated earlier (lines 97–121) about the left and right ventricular support options. He describes the two biventricular device options. The paracorporeal VAD option (PVAD-BiVAD) (lines omitted) is based on older technology, has "pumps hung outside the body, making the blood circulation visible." The more recent fully implantable pumps, the second and third generation nonpulsatile VADs, include the Heartware-HVAD. Dr. S describes the PVAD-BiVAD as a reliable 1990s technology that works very effectively and has been recently successfully implanted in a patient with Giant Cell Myocarditis as a bridge to transplantation. Dr. S refers to the same patient who Dr. D has referred to in Chapter 3 when suggesting that Mr Spencer could get in touch with her to discuss her experience. Then, Dr. S. describes the most recent technology of the Heartware-HVAD, which has been implanted and cleared by the FDA as an LVAD and could also be experimentally used as an RVAD. The right ventricle operation to insert the HVAD has never been done at this hospital, and it is not cleared by the FDA. However, special permission can be granted under a humanitarian device exemption, and a second HVAD can be implanted as right ventricular assist device support in Mr Spencer's chest. To follow the FDA guidelines ensuring maximum patient safety, this choice requires Dr. S to assemble a larger team to include personnel from the company that makes the HVAD. Both devices carry similar risks.

Dr. S. continues:

213	Dr. S:	they both carry similar risks
214		in terms of bleeding stroke uhhh
215		you know complications on the device uh
216		but I don't think there any there are any
217		there is no real elegant good easy out uh solution here
218		we were hoping and you know
219		you are at higher risk because of all the uhm
220		immunosuppressants you have been o:n
221		to try to combat this myocarditis
222		I do think it is it'll be helpful
223		to: sorta get you off of that before you
224		before a big surgery or operation

"There is no real elegant good easy out solution" (line 217). Mr Spencer will need to have a bridge to transplantation with either one of these two VADs options. Two major surgeries. Not an elegant, easy good solution. The implantation of these devices will require the healthcare team to temporarily remove Mr Spencer from the active heart transplantation waiting list until he has adequately recovered from this major surgery. As we previously discussed, Raia (2020) shows that AdHF healthcare professionals know that these experiences often provoke considerable anxiety in patients and their families for fear of not having recovered when the "right" heart becomes available. Not an elegant good easy-out solution. The experiences of learning to live tethered to a machine are challenging and complex (Kostick *et al.*, 2018, 2019; Raia & Deng, 2015b). The device is located partly inside and partly outside one's body and attached to batteries that need to be changed every 4 to 12 hours, and as Dr. S discusses, they have serious risks (lines 213–215). No, the implantation of these devices is not an elegant good easy solution.

Urgency-Related Tension in the Team

Mr Spencer is on a high dose of immunosuppressants to try to combat the disease (lines 220–221), reversing the Giant Cell Myocarditis and preserve Mr Spencer's heart. But now, the situation has changed, and this goal seems no longer achievable. With the newly formulated goal to prolong

Mr Spencer's life with BiVAD implantation as a bridge to transplantation, the immunosuppressive therapy makes no longer sense because it puts the patient at risk of infection as his immune competence, necessary to respond to infection, is depressed. Having a foreign body, the BiVAD in his body will make Mr Spencer more susceptible to infections even if he had not undergone immunosuppressant therapy. With the ongoing immunosuppressant treatment, this risk is steeply increased. Dr. S turns to the others on the team and asks about the dose of prednisone — an immunosuppressant:

overlaps

225	Dr. S:	where is prednisone right now by the way
226	Dr. D:	prednisone is at forty it think [right
227	RN. N:	[so it was at forty but uh thirty
228		uhm thirty six of solumedrol we've given
229	Dr. D:	uhm uhm
230	RN. N:	because we replaced it
231		because he had nausea [and vomiting
232	Dr. S:	[right
233	RN. N:	with these pills=
234	Dr. S:	=so what is the taper plan right now
235	RN. N:	right **now** we are not tapering
236	Dr. D:	Yea so we so we=
237	Dr. S:	=but if we're going to VA:D
238	Dr. D:	[then **yes**
239	Dr. S:	[I think we should start tapering [and
240	RN. N:	[yea::h
241	Dr. S:	[try to reduce the infectious risk
242	Dr. D:	[uhm uhm exactly right
243	Dr. S:	is what I'm concerned about
244	Dr. D	that's exactly right

It is the first time during this encounter that the participants talk over each other. To a hearer, it gives the impression of a brief but sudden tension — Dr. S's interruptions of CCU Nurse N (RN. N), the multiple overlaps (lines 226–227; 231–232; 238–239; 239–240; 241–242) of CCU Nurse N, Dr. S and Dr. D making similar points, gives the listener the impression that each of them competes in their role for the primary responsibility of initiating the immunosuppressant tapering. The coparticipant healthcare professionals create an interactional space from which Mr Spencer is excluded or, at best, is considered an overhearer. For example, at line 131, CCU Nurse N talks *about* Mr Spencer ("because he had nausea and vomiting").

Dr. D, in cogen session, discusses how "at this point, the situation could become problematic":

> Dr. S's insistence on tapering is particularly striking, especially when CCU Nurse N highlights that "we" are not tapering (line 235). This "we" does not include Dr. S but points to Dr. D and the AdHF Fellow responsible for the medical management. Mr. Spencer could understand this as an insight into a conflict of opinion or, worse, negligence: it is crucial to have trust from the patient perspective. That is why I say 'that is exactly right.' I do this all the time when I perceive the possibility that the patient can perceive our multidisciplinary decision-making processes as disagreement rather than our process of reaching a consensus on the best next steps.

After all, as Mr Spencer has pointed out, it is the New Year's Day, and the healthcare professionals had no chance to discuss the issue in their weekly meeting. This meeting described in Chapter 5 is the meeting the team calls the "Selection Committee" or simply "The Friday Meeting" because it is held each Friday at 7:00 a.m. Seventy-five multidisciplinary professionals are invited, as a selection committee, to discuss each case in detail and make decisions regarding therapeutic options. Not all need to attend each case. Usually, 30 to 40 professionals attend each meeting. Not today, though. Today is a holiday, and the professionals had not met to discuss Mr Spencer's case before the encounter.

Backstage and Frontstage Communication

While Dr. S and Mr Spencer and his family continue to talk, another parallel conversation among the other healthcare professionals present in the room unfolds. The AdHF Fellow asks Dr. D which immunosuppressant tapering protocol he prefers. Dr. D, also consulting with CCU Nurse N, decides the next steps for immunosuppressant medications (tacrolimus, mycophenolate, and methylprednisolone) of the tapering protocol tailored explicitly to Mr Spencer's current situation. These include dosing plans for the following days, as shown in Fig. 6.2, in which methylprednisolone dosing is changed for the next day and the day after it.

To make sense of the different kinds of communications spaces, we recall Goffman's model of social interaction (1959) introduced in Chapter 2. Goffman uses the metaphor of a theatrical performance to make sense of how humans conduct themselves in social life. He argues that humans enact particular roles for others who, in turn, play the part of the audience. Goffman's model distinguishes the "frontstage" performance for an audience from a "backstage" behavior where an actor might be alone or hidden from the audience's view and hearing. In medical interactions, if we assign the role of an audience to the patients and their families, utilizing Goffman's model of social interaction, we can identify the two regions. Frontstage, the shared region, where the actions of the practitioners are visible to the patient, and backstage, a remote region, in which the practitioners can refine their actions without being heard or seen by Mr Spencer and his family. In this model, Mr Spencer's room in CCU is a frontstage communication, and the morning meeting room, where the AdHF healthcare professionals usually discuss current patients' cases, is the backstage. Modeled this way, we can argue that during holiday time, the impossibility of discussing Mr Spencer's case during the backstage morning meeting had created the necessity to reach consensus among the healthcare professionals in frontstage, in Mr Spencer's room.

However, it is in Mr Spencer's room, after the brief overlapping of talk (lines 225–244) hinting at tension among the multidisciplinary team members, that the social organization of participants' behaviors changes fast.

FRONT STAGE		BACKSTAGE	
245	Dr S:	and it's not just the infection at the time of surgery alone (.)		
246		it can be the infectious risks weeks down the line (.8)		
247		when you start off immunosuppressed		
248		we just want		
249		uh to decrease that risk as well		
250		*SO* if we have **time** uh (.6)	AdHF F:	so what forty thirty
251		I think there are a couple benefits		twenty
252		first we want to start off		something like that
253		by getting you off some of these immunosuppressants		
254		which puts you at a higher procedural	Dr D:	yea I think it's

The apparent tension on lines 225 to 244 resolves quickly. The surgeon turns to address Mr Spencer again (line 245), and a parallel conversation — in the transcripts highlighted in gray — unfolds among the CCU Nurse N, the AdHF Fellow, and Dr. D.

The AdHF Fellow and the Nurse move both close to Dr. D to transform Dr. S's urgent request into practice instructions. Hindmarsh and Pilnick (2002), in their study of interprofessional communication in general surgery, extend Goffman's back/frontstage model to show that a backstage can be created as extempore space, e.g., by performing actions outside the patient's limited peripheral vision (p. 159). In their study, the patient's participation shifts from being copresent and overhearing conversations before anesthesia to being absent after anesthesia is administered. The teamwork during surgery, in turn, is described by the authors as progressively becoming more back region as the patient drifts off, and the transition between frontstage and backstage can be tracked alongside the patient's changing state of consciousness as the general anesthesia is administered. Raia and Smith (2020) extend the front/backstage model to study the communication patterns in the multiactivity practice of teaching and learning and patient care during the heart biopsy in the AdHF. In this situation, the AdHF Attending and the Nurse simultaneously teach the AdHF Fellow in training and care for the patient. The patient remains awake throughout the procedure and, therefore, is always at least potentially copresently aware of and monitoring the clinicians' talk. Raia and Smith find that creating extempore back and frontstages is a skill learned during AdHF training in practice. In Mr Spencer's CCU room, the coparticipant healthcare professionals create extempore back/front regions in the interaction of the medical practice. A backstage communication allows Dr. D, CCU Nurse N, and the AdHF Fellow to communicate about the tapering plan (reported in note Fig. 6.2). This region is also open to Dr. S. He is a ratified participant who can see and understand their consulting action on the current medication, as reflected in his talk (line 253).

FRONTSTAGE			BACKSTAGE	
255	Dr S:	but i don't want to uh put you in jeopardy in	AdHF F:	forty thirty twenty=
256		by having you have some event	Dr D:	=yeah
257		where we need to put you on ECMO to save your life	AdHF F:	and then what
258		and take two steps back before we start going forward again		keep the mycyphenolate keep tac
259		so its kinda of it's kind of a problem for us too to get you		what do you wanna do
260		the best outcome uh		keep the tac
261		RIGHT now you seem to be well		mycyphenolate is
262		perfused the numbers I see on your labs		at what dose right now
263		when I look at your *overall* (0.6) are	RN. N:	it's at one point five grams
264		reassuring from the standpoint of perfusion (0.8)	Dr D:	twice
265		but like I said I think you are on a very narrow edge here		twice or once
266		and one that could that can change and ((monitors loud beeps))	RN. N:	Twice
267		and you know you're talking to me	Dr D:	so we could downtitrate
268		you're asking very insightful questions		tac is at point five right? bid
269		and it's very clear you're all there	AdHF F:	uh uh
270		and and you have a lot life to live	Dr D:	go mycophenolate to thousand bid
271		you're young um		Continue tapering pred
272		I think we should go all in and and		and we Hold ritux obviously
273		and try to get you the best outcome		

The copresent Mr Spencer and his family are considered unratified members in the interactions in backstage between Dr. D, CCU Nurse N, and the AdHF Fellow. Even though the microphone is very close to where they are positioned, it is difficult to hear and understand their talk. They whisper and use elliptical language (M. H. Goodwin, 1996) that restricts an audience's accessibility by using talk comprehensible only to specialists. Interestingly, the Fellow's voice is more audible than those of both CCU Nurse N's and Dr. D's voices, although farthest away from the microphone. Both CCU Nurse N and Dr. D's utterances are whispered as if not wanting to interfere with the simultaneously ongoing frontstage dialogue. This more attentive and skillful practice of the Attending and Nurse is consistent with Raia and Smith's (2020) work on variation in communicative skills and their development during teamwork. We can also identify another motivation for the quick formation of an extempore back/frontstage resolving the tension: the urgency of the situation that dictates a well-coordinated back/frontstage performance in order "not to lose time."

The parallel conversation in frontstage continues. Mr Spencer, right now (line 261), seems to have good blood flow (perfused, line 262 and perfusion, line 264), as shown by his blood analysis (line 261) of kidney, liver, and metabolism functions. The team continually monitors blood pressure, heart rhythm, and blood oxygen saturation showing up on the monitors in the room. Mr Spencer's cognitive functions are stable, a symptom of good blood and oxygen circulation, as Dr. S points out, evaluating his capacity for making decisions. But, this is an urgent situation, and things can change as the possibility of going on ECMO looms like a sword of Damocles (lines 256–258); Mr Spencer is on a narrow edge (line 265). He is young and should opt to live (lines 269–272) by agreeing to the recommended options rather than wait when sudden precipitation of events can lead to the undesired solution: the not elegant solution of a bridge to a bridge.

Assigning agency

274	Mr. Spencer:	Today
275	Dr. S:	I don't think uh today is going to necessarily be the day
276		just because of the logistics

Is this happening "today"? Mr Spencer asks. Dr. S takes "this" to refer to the machine implantation surgery. He will need to assemble the team. The logistics (line 276) involved in organizing for either implantation option — the Heartware-HVAD not approved by FDA for both the left and the right ventricles, or the "reliable 1990's technology" (line 174) omitted — are different. Which one Dr. S will organize depends on the result of the shared decision-making process developing right now in Mr Spencer's room.

277	Dr. S:	and like I said
278		if you give us a little time to get some of these drugs off
279		and make you a better candidate
280		I think there'd be benefit now
281		if you start to show a little more lability
282		like your you go back in and out of Vtach umm
283		or your your numbers start to show that your perfusion
284		your kidney your liver are starting to suffer
285		and we follow that very closely
286		then I would say we do it right there and then

"if you give us a little time." Dr. S uses the transitive verb (to give) positioning Mr Spencer as an agent who acts on the object, the team: if Mr Spencer can "give a little time" to the team to get him off the immunosuppressants, if Mr Spencer can give a little time to the team to make him better. This sentence is a change from the previous talk in which the surgeon has explained what could happen and what the team would do to Mr Spencer. Here, Mr Spencer gives time to the team. Whether Dr. S is conscious or not of how he is framing it, the wording frames Mr Spencer as an active agent in the process (lines 278–281). However, Mr Spencer does not have the power to do this action.

Mindful that "stating is performing an act" (Austin, 1965, p. 138), it is relevant to call on Duranti's work (2005) on how agency is enacted (e.g., assigned, mitigated, or negated) and represented in language: Agency is "understood as the property of those entities (i) that have some degree of control over their own behavior, (ii) whose actions in the world affect other entities' (and sometimes their own), and (iii) whose actions are the object of evaluation (e.g., in terms of their responsibility for a given outcome)" (p. 451).

If we focus on the first two criteria of Duranti's working definition, we can say that Dr. S recognizes Mr Spencer's agency. He ascribes the capacity of action and some degree of control over (i) Mr Spencer's own behavior (ii) and others, the team. However, the third criterion requires that Mr Spencer's actions are subject to evaluation, and Mr Spencer is responsible for giving or not giving time to the team to save his life. In studying physiotherapy interactions, Parry (2018) argues that both patients and therapists attribute agency to body parts with the effect of deflecting responsibility for something out of their control. Dr. S's utterance attributing agency to Mr Spencer would point to and be consistent with Dr. S's previously expressed concerns of Mr Spencer being on a razor's edge (lines 31–40). Something out of his and the team's control: a ventricular tachycardia (v-tach, line 282) event that can degenerate into a lethal arrhythmia and degradation of other organ functions (lines 283–284). These adverse events require the urgent implantation of ECMO (lines 41–45), but they can also turn into Mr Spencer's death. In this interpretation, allocating agency to Mr Spencer has the effect of mitigating the responsibility for things that are out of D S's and the team's control. However, irrespective of Dr. S's intention, it also has another potential, a detrimental consequence for Mr Spencer. He can feel blamed and responsible for something out of his control.

What Dr. S and the team can do, however, is to monitor the situation very closely (line 285), and what Dr. S, in particular, can do is to give medical advice (line 285). Mr Spencer calls Dr. D from backstage and asks whether he is on the list (question 1, line 289).

287	Mr. Spencer:	Dr. D
288	Dr. D:	Yes
289	Mr. Spencer:	am I on the*list*
290	Dr. D:	I think-so
291		we're closing the uhh the ad hoc mechanism
292		and you will be therefore on the list uh very soon
293		formally that is a process-that-is happening now

Mr Spencer's QUESTION (lines 287–289)

Dr. D responds by describing the process that is currently unfolding to accept Mr Spencer on the list. The ad hoc mechanism (line 291) described in Chapter 5, initiated by Dr. D, is about to conclude; the formal process of communicating Mr Spencer's name to the UNOS list for heart transplantation is most probably almost complete. Indeed, while all 75 members of the committee receive the information, the relevant decision-makers — AdHF Attending cardiologist, Dr. D, AdHF surgeon assigned to the patient, Dr. S, the surgical and medical directors of the transplant program, infection disease specialist, psychiatrist, nurse specialists, social worker, and pharmacist — have already agreed.

294	Dr. D:	and uh what Dr. S' outlining is linking basically
295		it's the other you know starting point of view
296		that we've been discussing
297		the last days to be prepared for this option
298		and uhm including the different
299		mechanical options that we discussed uhm
300		and including a timeline that is sooner rather than later
301		uhm so right now it's what
302		coming back to what we have discussed in these days
303		to uh detail the plan and as Dr. S says

304	between these two options
305	mainly of biventricular assist over the next days
306	this is all under the assumption
307	from ours and the arrhythmia team's perspective
308	that this is all stable
309	and as you see there is some movement with the arrhythmia
310	so we want to be prepared for the step uh
311	to proceed any time
312	that's why we have have what's
313	while we are having the conversation right now you know
314	(6.0)

Dr. D links (294) his answer to Mr Spencer's question to what Dr. S has discussed about the two options of a bridge to transplantation (lines 298–299). He organizes the discussion in a timeline (starting at line 300), which includes three points: (1) Dr. D's and Mr Spencer's past days' conversation about possible options (line 302). Until now, those were quite remote possibilities; today, they had to become part of the solution (line 305) for Mr Spencer to remain alive. (2) The development Dr. S has been discussing with Mr Spencer. Dr. D refers to Dr. S explicitly naming him (lines 294 and 303). (3) In reference to the team (line 307), Dr. D includes himself in it, saying, "we want to be prepared" (line 310), clearly pointing to a team effort and agreement. However, while talking to Mr Spencer, Dr. D also notices some short episode of arrhythmia (line 309) that fortunately seems to dissipate quickly.

315	Mr. Spencer:	and so at any given any time	Mr. Spencer's QUESTION
316		even in the ni**ght** (.)	
317		there is a (2.0)	
318		experienced team that is assembled to do it if it happens	
319	Dr. D:	yes	
320	Mr. Spencer:	doesn't catch [us	
321	Dr. D:	[YES	
322	Mr. Spencer:	by [surprise	
323	Dr. D:	[YES	
324	Dr. S:	[yes same team	

Dr. S's previous answers have resolved Mr Spencer's doubt about the quality of the team during holidays and a 24-hour cycle so, a short response "Yes. Same team," "Yes" puts this doubt to rest, and Mr Spencer moves on to the next question:

325	Mr. Spencer:	if uh (1.4)	Mr. Spencer's QUESTION
326		if I get umm the ventricular assist (1.0) things (1.0)	
327		does that put me lower on the list? because then I have a bridge	
328	Dr. D:	So so the important thing here (0.7)	
329		is all under the big (.) picture question	
330		what gives Mr. Spencer	
331		the highest likelihood to go to the age of one hundred fifty two	
332		and help his wife do the *dish*es at the age one hundred fifty two	
333		which is your ultimate quality of life	
334		comparing the different options	
335		Ongoing-medical-therapy-including-immunosuppression *(faster pace))*	
336		may not be (.) the *best ((slower pace))*	
337		number *two:*	
338		listing for heart transplantation *YES*	
339		Number *three:*	
340		while waiting may need mechanical support uh	
341		in order *to* get to transplantation (.) *yes*	
342		and part of this option is after mechanical-support	
343		during-a-couple-of-weeks of-recovery-from-that surgery *(faster pace))*	
344		you are changed from highest urgency to transplant	
345		to temporarily non-transplantable	
346		and then active on the list again	
347		and the urgency status will be the unos *one*	
348		it will be likely one *B* uh first	
349		and there's some options of one *A* as-well?	
350		so that is not the key	
351		uh you know the decision maker here	
352		the main question is to *saf*ely get (1.) *to* transplantation (.)	
353		uhh (.6) in a meaningful way	
354		that's what we are preparing for right now	
355		and the right question asked uhh	
356		with a twenty four seven preparedness	
357		that is the important thing (2.)	

Does the bridge to transplantation put Mr Spencer lower on the transplant list (lines 326–327)? Dr. D reframes the question. It is not a step back from being on UNOS 7. It is a necessary step within the "big picture" (line 329) goal of living a long and good quality life (line 333) with transplantation. Note that the pause after "big (.)," on line 329, creates a short suspension in the utterance augmenting the importance of words "big (.) picture." Dr. D plays on what he perceives as a typical family life situation of asking "who does the dishes?" and refers to it jokingly as a loving moment. At line 323, subtle laughter is audible from the back of the room where Mr Spencer's family is standing. Dr. D continues by using a similar speech pattern on line 336. This time the emphasis given to the words "may not be (.) the *best*" is accentuated by a faster speech rate (fast pace) on line 335, accompanied by a slower speech rate and the emphasis on the word "*best.*" Dr. D continues by highlighting the steps taken so far in the shared decision-making process, recapitulating them ("number two, number three options"; lines 338–339).

Similarly to what we saw in Chapter 3, the doctor creates a temporal horizon (Raia, 2020): he first grounds Mr Spencer in a common existential past, which is relatively recent in terms of clock time, just a few days, but existentially very significant as Mr Spencer's life has been changing dramatically. Dr. D calls upon their common existential past by pointing to their critical discussions preparing for these changes in Mr Spencer's life a few days prior (lines 296–297). Then, Dr. D projects Mr Spencer into future possibilities of being with his wife. Grounding Mr Spencer in a shared past and projecting him into the future possibility of being himself, Dr. D can reframe the question and current understanding of the "big picture" (line 329) (Raia, 2020).

It is interesting to note that Dr. D (line 334) says: "comparing the different options." as shown in Chapter 3, the way AdHF doctors discuss the options follows a different logical sequence: Option 1, guidelines directed medical therapy that excludes surgeries (e.g., immunosuppressants to reverse the myocarditis and restore native heart function); Option 2, heart transplant; Option 3, lifetime mechanic support. Here, Dr. D is not following this abstract decision-making algorithm because he is not talking in general about the therapeutic options. He describes them in the specificity of the situation. He has framed them for Mr Spencer from the beginning of their interactions and emerging as necessary in Mr Spencer's current life situation.

On lines 344 to 349, Dr. D returns to Mr Spencer's question about being lowered on the UNOS status list (line 327) but is also mindful of Mr Spencer's question of being on the list at all (line 289). In cogen session, we discussed the issue of thinking about the UNOS listing as "active" and "non-active" listing for transplantation. These terms are misleading. Indeed the patient remains listed on the UNOS list in both cases because s/he has already been evaluated and approved for transplantation. However, a misleading colloquial way of talking about the change of status from any active listing status (UNOS 1 through 6) to nonactive (UNOS 7 Temporarily non-Transplantable) translates into using the terms "off the list" or "de-listed" without specifying the difference between active and nonactive listing. This imprecise and careless talk can induce anxiety in patients for the unfounded but perceived fear of been abandoned by the team as no longer a good candidate for transplantation.

Mr Spencer's decision. No ghoulish options

Mr Spencer's
DECISION

358	Mr. Spencer:	uhm (1.6)
359		I don't want (.) stuff hanging outside of my body
360		when t's done (.)
361	Dr. S:	so=
362	Mr. Spencer:	=I WOULD go:: for an electrical thing
363		the the vtach? or even two of them
364		with a place to plug them in and charge it
365	Dr. D:	uhm uhm
366	Mr. Spencer:	but*external* devices that (0.9) are pumping my heart
367		and things like that (0.6)
368		I don't want to go that far (5)
		((creeky voice))
369	Dr. D:	That would be hvad bivad
370		as opposed to pvad bivad
371	Mr. Spencer:	O:r an artificial heart (0.9)
372	Dr. D:	and say that sentence of the artificial heart again
373		because we discussed that three days ago
374	Mr. Spencer:	No
375	Dr. D:	O:key a no okay [I get it
376	Mr. Spencer:	[So basically uhmm
377		either this heart makes it to the transplant or
378		you use ventricular devices or device
379		to get me there
380	Dr. D:	uh uh
381	Mr. Spencer:	or you let me go
382	Dr. D:	uh uh
383	Mr. Spencer:	I don't think I've heard of any other options that are (1.)
384		uhmm (3.5) not ghoulish (1.7)
385	Dr. D:	You are ri::ght these are the main uhm (2.)

Mr Spencer does neither want any form of visual of his blood being pumped outside his body nor an artificial heart; he does not see any other solution that is not ghoulish.

Mr Spencer's doubt

Dr. D remains in silence, meaningfully acknowledging the importance of Mr Spencer's decision. There is nothing to be added to that. However, Dr. S picks up on the doubt in Mr Spencer's utterance on line 383: "I don't think I've heard of any other options," because he responds to it, trying to reassure Mr Spencer.

386	Dr. S:	It's you know the:: (1.2)
387		the first time you are confronted with the:se?
388		it's just an enormous emotional toll in my opinion and
389		I've done this conversation enough to know that
390		what you are going through right now
391		is not unique? (0.6)
392		you have to (1.0) get (0.5)
393		kinda wrap your mind around this idea
394		of of these artificial devices and
395		what they represent (0.7) umm
396		I understand ANYbody's aversion
397		to having things hanging outside their body pumping blood that is
398		that doesn't sound like in any way tolerable at all (0.7) um
399		it is the wa:=
400		that up until four five years ago the ma*jor*ity of patients
401		who did get to transplant with devices were do:ne and
402		they got there but
403		we have other OPTIOns now in [year] and
404		I and I don't disagree with you?
405		I just want you to be *awa*re and
406		as long as you und*erstan*d that
407		it is not FDA approved for that side? um
408		but people are using them that way?
409		and getting people to transplant? uhm
410		then I think that's all I need to hear from you:
411		you are very insightful and
412		you are very clear right now with what you want so
413		I I feel with great conviction
414		you are making the decision that you feel is appropriate
415	Mr. Spencer:	And you understand what (0.9) what I've said
416	Dr. S:	yes
417	Mr. Spencer:	as far as (1.0)
418	Dr. D:	uh uh

419	Mr. Spencer:	how far I am willing to go
420	Dr. S:	Yes
421	Mr. Spencer:	Okay

Mr Spencer's doubt does not come from the emotional toll (line 388) of accepting what these artificial devices represent (line 395) in a person's life. It comes from the question of "you understand what (0.9) what I've said? (line 415). For Mr Spencer, the important existential decision is: do nothing ghoulish (line 419). I accept death. Mr Spencer pushes Dr. S to understand and accept the existential dimension independently of the technological option available in high-tech medicine. Dr. S's "yes" on line 416 is barely audible compared to his other utterances as if humbled in the face of accepting death as part of life.

Dr. D takes on the conversation to finalize the plan, reach a consensually shared decision, and complete the consent signing.

422	Dr. D:	There is one one one uhh
423		ad thought that I want to share
424		let's assume next twenty four hours
425		you are on the highest urgency waiting list and
426		assume that the arrhythmias are stable uh
427		((beeping sound from heart monitor for sudden arrhythmias))

The sudden loud monitor alarm showing the heart rate of 190 beats per minute is unmistakable for all in the room. Another code blue?

CHAPTER 7

TRANSITIONING FROM URGENCY TO EMERGENCY: THE ROLE OF THE EXISTENTIAL DIMENSION

We concluded the last chapter when Dr. D was stating the premise of his reasoning "let's assume that the arrhythmias are stable" (line 426). Ironically, the loud piercing sound of the heart monitoring system alerted the room on the onset of new episodes of arrhythmias (line 427); we report it again below. A passage from an urgency to an emergency introduces a change of pace, risk, and uncertainty. The recommendations and the ensuing discussions with Mr Spencer and his family within a shared decision-making process that relies on legal, ethical, and clinical dimensions, as discussed in Chapter 3, must be addressed in a dynamic, time-dependent frame, creating a more complex situation (Joseph-Williams *et al.*, 2014; Légaré *et al.*, 2008; Pieterse *et al.*, 2019; Raia *et al.*, 2021; Rotenstein *et al.*, 2017).

The episodes of arrhythmia dissipating quickly earlier (Chapter 6, line 309) are starting again.

428	Dr. D:	There is one one one uhh
429		ad thought that I want to share
430		let's *assu*me next twenty four hours
431		you are on the highest urgency waiting list
432		and *assu*me that the arrhythmias are stable uh
433		*BEE:::::P BEE:::::P BEE:::::P*
		((beeping sound from heart monitor for sudden arrhythmias))
434		which uh may not be the case
		BEE:::::P BEE:::::P BEE:::::P
435		Uhm then we can wait for the heart
		BEE:::::P BEE:::::P BEE:::::P
436		uhm uh for these next short time periods days=
437	Dr. S:	=did you just feel something just now
438	Mr Spencer:	I did a little like a little bump

147

"let's a*ssu*me" there is stability (line 430); Dr. D repairs the sentence (line 426) with "which uh may not be the case" (line 428). He treads carefully not to exclude the possibility of waiting for a few days to see whether a heart offer arrives while preparing for Biventricular Assist Device (BiVAD) implantation (lines 433–436).

With the arrhythmia developments, Dr. D will need to introduce an additional step: an emergency Extracorporeal Membrane Oxygenator (ECMO) might become necessary as a bridge to the BiVAD implantation. Dr. S, who was inspecting the monitor, jumps into the conversation, latching into Dr. D's talk (line 437). Did Mr Spencer feel the ventricular tachycardia (v-tach)? He did; "a little bump" (line 438). The alarms continue marking Mr Spencer's v-tach, his heart at 190 beats/min. There is a good chance that this unstable v-tach can degenerate into lethal ventricular fibrillation (v-fib). Dr. D resumes his talk:

439	Dr. D:	yeah and if it's not stable and uhm
440		we are preparing for the mechanical support uhm
441		the preparation for the HVAD the uhm
442		implantable device just takes a bit=
443	Dr. S:	=a little bit
444	Dr. D:	and=
445	Dr. S:	=lem*me* ask you one thing uhm
446		if you do need to go on ECMO though
447		just to get to a safe place to get you to the VAD
448		would you have any issue with that
449		cause that's not a
450		that's something we need to address right now

Dr. D's talk is in stark contrast to the loud beeping sound of the alarm; he proceeds slowly, as if the situation, turning into a possible emergency, does not affect him. He takes Mr Spencer through the steps toward the prospect of needing an ECMO, pointing to the time it takes to prepare for BiVAD implantation surgery. It "just takes a bit" (line 442), but Dr. S intervenes (lines 443 and 445). As if in a relay race, he picks up the "bit" from Dr. D and runs with it. First, with a calm but inadequately casual tone ("would you have any issue with that," line 448), not to alarm Mr Spencer, he presents the prospect of an ECMO implantation that he previously referred to as a "setback" (line 45, Chapter 6).[1] Now the ECMO is something "just"

---

[1] Dr. S has described the ECMO during the same encounter (lines 46–53; Chapter 6).

to get Mr Spencer to a safe place (line 447) as if a simple decision on a preference and not on a significant component of life support can be made by Mr Spencer. Then, with a sharp acceleration, Dr. S asks for immediate verbal consent ("right now," line 450). The situation is escalating. Everybody can feel it in the room with the incessant beeping from the heart monitor.

Both Dr. D and Dr. S worry that Mr Spencer, who has an aversion to medically excessive interventions, will not be able to come to terms with and agree to an ECMO in the very short-time window that could present if he goes into v-fib.

In cogen, Dr. S reflects on the passage:

Dr. S: "you're constantly surveying a situation. At the beginning of this conversation, Mr Spencer was discussing with me, and his vitals were stable. But with the occurrence of these events, you realize that the situation is changing. Mr Spencer may arrest. You feel the urgency in my tone."

Mr Spencer could code, leaving the physicians with only a slim opportunity to save his life.

Professional Visions

In his seminal paper, *professional vision*, C. Goodwin (1994) demonstrates that the perceptions and understanding of events "are not idiosyncratic phenomena restricted to individuals but shared frameworks, domain of professional competence. [...] Socially organized ways of seeing and understanding events are answerable to the distinctive interests of a particular social group making up the work environment of a scientific discipline." In addition to studying the production and use of graphic representations (e.g., Coopmans *et al.*, 2014; Lynch & Woolgar, 1990), Goodwin (1994) proposes to analyze the professional competencies by looking at what the professionals *highlight* as salient and what they *code*, i.e., "transforming phenomena observed into the objects of knowledge that animate the discourse of a profession." Utilizing Goodwin's work, we can identify in the current interactions the "socially organized ways of seeing and understanding events" that make up the Advanced Heart Failure (AdHF) profession's specific competence in practice. For example, as the event unfolds (lines 422–444), Dr. D operates a self-repair on line 434, showing that what has just happened is relevant enough to modify what he has been discussing with Mr Spencer (*highlighting*). Dr. S highlights the same phenomenon, intervening in the conversation and asking Mr Spencer about his perception of the v-tach (line 437). The alarm's loud beeping, the changing tempo produced by the heart monitor marking the fast heartbeats, and the hemodynamic graphical display are categorized and understood by the AdHF professionals in the room as the onset of v-tach. They all *code* the situation as very urgent with the possibility of degenerating into an emergency.

The two professionals highlight the same phenomenon and code it similarly. However, they act differently. Dr. D, the AdHF cardiologist, after a self-repair (line 434) treads very carefully in his talk to Mr Spencer, while Dr. S, the AdHF surgeon, moves for immediate consent for the procedure (line 450). The question we raise here is: are those idiosyncratic reactions restricted to individuals' responses to a situation moving from urgency to emergency, or are those the resulting actions of specific competencies of each professional in their own domain of expertise, e.g., AdHF surgery and AdHF cardiology, and therefore marking two distinct professional visions?

As we proceed with the encounter, we show that, with the same *highlighting* and *coding*, we need to add the action each professional will have to take to make sense of Dr. D's and Dr. S's conduct. We call this new element for the analysis *anticipated actions*. *Highlighting* and *coding* manifest the meaning-making actions in the present situation. However, as discussed in Chapter 2, Raia (2018, 2020) demonstrates that the actions we take and the situations we face are not only intelligible to us but matter to us, allowing our emotional investment in the activities manifesting in how we partake in them. In Raia's framework, what Goodwin points to as professional *highlighting* emerges from a process of learning that goes beyond what is intelligible. It is a process of *becoming* a professional that is rooted in the person's past experiences and, at the same time, projected in the future possibility of being this person, this professional, e.g., Dr. S.

Within this framework, we do not need to consider emotional responses as an add-on to meaning-making because emotional responses and stances, such as the feeling of urgency Dr. S recognized in his tone, are part of being a professional for whom matters what is happening. For Dr. S, caring for Mr Spencer and "returning him to his family" is what matters. To do so, Dr. S is anticipating different actions (*anticipated actions*) he has already shared with Mr Spencer earlier in the encounter (Chapter 6). Dr. S will need to take these actions as soon as he walks out of Mr Spencer's room to do the surgery by the evening. Indeed, as described in Chapter 6, the Heartware-VAD has been utilized and cleared by the United States Food and Drug Administration (FDA) only as a Left Ventricular Assist Device (LVAD). It has neither been implanted at this hospital nor cleared by the FDA to support the heart's right ventricle. Dr. S will need to obtain special permission granted under a humanitarian device exemption to experimentally use it as a Right Ventricular Assist Device (RVAD). To follow the FDA guidelines ensuring maximum patient safety, Dr. S needs to assemble a larger team to include personnel from the company that makes the HeartWare BiVAD (HVAD). Dr. S and Dr. D reflect in cogen:

> Dr. S: In the back of my mind, I'm thinking this is a big undertaking. It could go awry. This could be terrible, it's the first one[2], and I'm advocating for something which I'd never done before. You know, we're going to do the best we can, which is bringing in the support of people who've seen it done before and can guide us and proctor us through this process. [...] As a surgeon, you have to figure out all this and have to figure out how to portrait? confidence, but not cockiness, being upfront and forthright with the patient; confidence with full disclosure.
>
> Dr. D: My task is to deliver the patient to the surgical team in a meaningful way, that is, with an authentic decision made. Then I go home and have a glass of wine with my wife. Yes, it is really like the metaphor of the relay we discussed. Dr. S takes up from here. He calls home and says I'm not gonna be home tonight because I'm gonna spend the next eight hours in the operating room. So that's exactly how it feels.

---

[2]Dr. S has informed Mr Spencer that the procedure has never been done at this hospital.

A Bridge to a Bridge to Transplantation

ECMO to VAD? Mr Spencer probes deeper:

451	Mr. Spencer:	ECMO to the VAD
452		that would be all within the same **room**
453		within the same ti:me
454	Dr. S:	well what we'd
455		no it would not it would be
456		ECMO would be done **her**e a:nd
457		we would put in the cannulas in he:re at the beside or
458		maybe even the surgical ICU? and then uhm
459		we would have uh you on that for a day or **two**
460		before we went to VAD
461		so it's uh that's=
462	Mr. Spencer:	=three three procedures to get to a heart transplant
463	Dr. S:	It *is* it's a it's a bridge to a bridge so to speak

If ECMO is necessary, Mr Spencer counts the three procedures, ECMO, VAD implantation, and heart transplantation; Dr. S reformulates them as one continuum (*framing*): a bridge to a bridge to heart transplantation, and at the same time, caring for Mr Spencer, orienting him toward a definitive therapy, heart transplantation.

464	Dr. S:	it's it's
465		but if you if something happens to you and
466		your heart stops? and people are doing CPR?
467		one of the options to try to get you out of it?
468		chemically and with chest compressions? uh and
469		hope that you come back? and
470		the other option-if those don't and
471		then **withdra**w if things are not going the way that
472		we want them to:?
473	Mr. Spencer:	o:r
474	Dr. S:	or we put you on ECMO and
475		that gives you a little bit of uh of **time** (.)

The situation can escalate, Dr. S continues: if his heart stops and Mr Spencer needs to be resuscitated, one option is to try Cardiopulmonary Resuscitation (CPR), heart compression with defibrillation (i.e., electric shocks), and/or by chemical resuscitation using inotropes and vasopressor drugs. But then stop (withdraw, line 465) if there is no response. Or? Asks Mr Spencer. "Or we put you on ECMO."

Consenting for ECMO: "The nuclear option"

Dr. S continues:

476	Dr. S:	but ECMO you know
477		it would go through the le:g? it would be uh
478		you know it would be a
479		proce-another procedure as you said uh
480		it's it's a
481		you it's a circuit with blood coming out
482		it goes to the pump and then comes back to your body
483		is that something you would be amenable to
484		or or not=
485	Mr. Spencer:	=only if it was part of the same procedure you were doing it
486		while you got me set up for the VAD and
487		when I came out it was (.) on=
488	Dr. S:	=no it's a separate procedure

Mr Spencer had often discussed his reservation against excessive interventions to save his life, as he did with his wife when he overheard the electrical shocks and the incessant pounding to resuscitate a patient next door to him in the CCU: "how far do we go as Christians to scratch and claw at hanging on to this life when we know that this world is not our home?" (Chapter 3, segment 3.1). The ECMO implantation is for him an extra procedure, to get to transplantation, and one too many:

489	Mr. Spencer:	no that's that's *three* (1.0) open heart (.) surgeries=
490	Dr. S:	=it's-not-open-heart
491		it goes through your groin (0.8)
492		we do it through the groin uhm
493	Mr. Spencer:	the pump hangs out of my leg
494	Dr. S:	the the *cannu*las hang out
495		the pumps-at-the-bedside are much like your uh
496		looks something you know
497		like something like this size right here it it
498		I'm not so sure on ECMO you would even be aware it's there (.)

As if to plug gushing water, Dr. S rushes to utter the words ("= it's-not-open-heart" (line 490) and amends Mr Spencer's understanding that ECMO is another open heart surgery (line 489). But the pumps would be hanging out of his body, Mr Spencer retorts. The cannulae, rectifies Dr. S, will be visible hanging out. Rushing the words "pumps-at-the-bedside," Dr. S moves to show how small the pumps are to revise Mr Spencer's perception.

But maybe more is needed to convince Mr Spencer that undergoing the ECMO procedure is essential to have a longer life with his family. Dr. S, as he commented in cogen, needs "a nuclear option":

499	Dr. S:	*okay* okay
500		let me let me just give you a suggestion cause uh
501		i'm a father and a husband *too* uhm (.)
502		it would
503		it could get you to the point
504		where you could get the VAD to the transplant(3.0)
505		and think of your family *too:* when you make this decision
506	Wife	ple:ase
		(6.0)
507	Dr. D:	maybe uh you uh
508		also want to talk about this uh for a [moment
509	Brother:	[(*(inaudible)*) of us too (0.6)
510		please agree to it (2.0)

Dr. D supports Dr. S's move and calls on the family to speak more.

Another Professional Vision in the Room

As shown below, the conversation continues with Dr. S clarifying that the reason why he wants Mr Spencer to accept the possibility of an ECMO procedure is not that Mr Spencer is unstable (lines 515, 517), but because of the complex preparation to initiate the HVAD BiVAD implantations surgery (lines 518–529). However, unexpectedly for Dr. S, Dr. D, Mr Spencer, and his family, the ECMO team enters the room (line 530). As the doctors try to ease Mr Spencer into accepting the possibility of a bridge to a bridge to transplantation for the ongoing consenting process, Mr Spencer is wary of any excessive and "futile" high-tech procedures to save his life. Although Mr Spencer is currently stable, as Dr. S clarifies (lines 515–517) in response to Mr Spencer's question (lines 511–512), the ensuing v-tach comports a higher probability of deterioration within the time Dr. S needs to assemble the team for surgery. The appearance of the ECMO team could not have happened at a worse time. The team unexpectedly arrives in the middle of a very delicate shared decision-making process. Its arrival could suggest that Dr. S and Dr. D are not taking into account Mr Spencer's strong reservation for ECMO implantation. Indeed, the entrance of the ECMO team would indicate that Mr Spencer is not stable. The ECMO team is usually called in emergency cases when a patient has coded already and either had previously consented to an ECMO procedure or had not been able to consent. However, Mr Spencer "is talking to us," Dr. S insists (lines 528, 534, and 541).

511	Mr. Spencer:	right now I'm not stable enough to get a VAD
512		is that what you're saying
513	Dr. S:	no no we're not
514	Dr. D:	no
515	Dr. S:	it has nothing to do with stabi*li*ty it has
516		you're talking to me
517		I can see you're stable
518		it it has everything to do with (.) the device selection and
519		getting you into the process (.)
520		uhm (.) and (.)
521		hopefully we can go: relatively quickly uh (1.0)
522		these are big undertakings I
523		you know I have to assemble not just ***our*** team but
524		I have to assemble the ***out***side team
525		that comes in too that helps manage these devices-it-is
526		and as I ***said***
527		the right sided device is not something that
528		we have a lot of experience with
		((ECMO team enters))
529		because it just hasn't been used for that
		((ECMO team talks to CCU Nurse N in the background))
530		[it's it's like using uh
531	ECMO Team:	[*((inaudible))*
532		[it's it's it's
533	ECMO Team:	[we need shock him out of it
534	Dr. S:	he's ***TAlk***ing to us
		((turns to ECMO team))
535	ECMO M1:	just a second let us take a look at here
536	ECMO M2:	I think we should have art-line
537	ECMO M3:	yea
538	ECMO M2:	just so you we know
539	ECMO M1:	yeah
540	Dr. S:	***but*** he's ***TALK***ing to us ***real***ly
541	ECMO M2:	I just gonna ATP him
542		*((inaudible))*
543		is this the most recent pressure for the cycle
544	RN. N:	I just did one
545		I'll do another one
546	Dr. S:	Look at the heart wave form he clearly perfuses
547		he is talking

548		he said some sentences with this pressure
549	ECMO M2:	I don't think you wanna (.) leave him in this
550	Mr Spencer:	hrh hrh ((clears his throat))
551	ECMO M3:	Did it just start now
552	AdHF Fellow:	yeah while we were talking about it
553	Dr. D:	Uh uh
554	ECMO M3:	Are you guys scaring him?
555	ECMO M2:	eh eh
556	Dr. S:	No he had the
557	Dr. D:	I think we are scaring you
558	Mr Spencer:	no:hh ((crying))

With the entrance of the ECMO team, the speakers' orientation changes from speaking *to* Mr Spencer to speaking to the ECMO team *about* Mr Spencer. (e.g., Mr Spencer "is talking to us," Dr. S insists, lines 534, 540, and 547). In contrast to Chapter 6, where a remote region (backstage) developed when the practitioners needed to refine their actions in order not to interfere with the conversation between Dr. S, Mr Spencer, and his family, in this situation, all participants will have access to the talk with the ECMO team. To show this change, rather than creating two parallel conversions as we did in Chapter 6, we underlined the ECMO team members and those speaking to them (second columns in the transcript).

In Goodwin's words, the ECMO team brings another professional vision into the scene of caring for Mr Spencer. From an ECMO team's perspective, the world looks like a potential emergency waiting for an ECMO to be implanted. The team entrance in Mr Spencer's room confers an emergency character to the situation that would require to shock Mr Spencer to restore his heart rhythm (line 533). The team moves to place an arterial line (artline line 536) and initiate an Anti-Tachycardia Pacing (ATP, line 541). At the same time, the ECMO team needs to acknowledge that Dr. S is correct; something must be stable and not an emergency requiring the three actions (lines 533, 536, and 541) to be taken immediately. Dr. S repeats three times that Mr Spencer "is *TALK*ing to us" (line 534), "*but* he's *TALK*ing to us *real*ly" (line 540), "he is talking" (line 547), indeed Mr Spencer did not code! "Look at the heart wave" urges Dr. S to the ECMO team, interpreting it as a sign of good perfusion (line 546).

In this interaction, Mr Spencer and his family are treated as unratified speakers by the ECMO team. Dr. S, who needs to demonstrate to the ECMO team that Mr Spencer did neither code nor is necessarily on the way to code, is compelled to talk *about* Mr Spencer in Mr Spencer's and his family's presence in the *frontstage*. Finally, the ECMO team initiates a playful "are you guys scaring him?" (line 554). Dr. D, rather than responding to the ECMO team, transforms the question to address Mr Spencer. He addresses Mr Spencer as a ratified speaker "I think we are scaring you" (line 557). Dr. D decomposes and reuses the communication resources by the ECMO team. This transformation has been shown by Goodwin (2018) to be pervasive in the organization of human action. In this instance, this cooperative action (C. Goodwin, 2018) has the essential function of facilitating the creation of two spaces of action, *back*, and *frontstages*. *Backstage*, the ECMO team continues talking with Dr. S and CCU Nurse N. In *frontstage*, Dr. D talks to Mr Spencer and his family. With the final separation of the spaces of communication, the pronoun "we" changes from "we," the hospital's teams, "are scaring you," Mr Spencer (line 557) into indicating "we", Mr Spencer *and* the AdHF team, "we have decisions in place" (line 561):

559	Dr. D:	I would think that would be part of the situation
560		the important thing is
561		we have decisions in place
562		on the listing now that'll be formalized
563		number two
564		we have a decision in place of biventricular assist device
565		that should be, if possible HVAD BiVAD
566		what we're right now discussing is
567		the ti:*me* to assemble everything will take so:me
568		and if we don't have the *time* uh
569		we have right now available a PVAD BiVAD but
570		those hang out of the body:
571		you have a statement in place that you don't want tha:t
572		we have
573		if more urgently bridging to either of these two
574		a VA-ECMO required currently a *thou*ght that uh
575		you would not want that
576		uhm this is by the way
577		the VA-ECMO is not the type of assist heart pump surgery
578		that of size of a uhm mechanical support or heart transplant
579		it's mo:re as we call it a *big* catheter based uh approach
580		So it's this uh
581		it doesn't have the same quality and
582		it's only for a few da:ys *to* uh have that longer term pump in place and
583		that would be an important in my opinion
584		a very favorable decision to make to uh uh to accept that

585   but uhm just from my perspective
586   it's not the same like three uh stage to heart transplant
587   it's um [VA-ECMO you know
                    [BE:::::
        BE:::::   BE::::   BE::::

From lines 561 to 579, Dr. D uses the pronoun "we" to include Mr Spencer, his family, and the AdHF team to summarize all the decisions made (i.e., lines 561, 564, 566, 568, and 572). First, to accept heart transplantation ("being on the list," line 562). "Number two" (line 563), the decision to have a bridge to transplantation via BiVAD. Rather than having visual access to the blood rotating into the pumps, which Mr Spencer would have if he had chosen the Paracorporeal Ventricular Assist Devices (PVAD) BiVAD implantation, Mr Spencer prefers the HVAD BiVAD because the actual pumps are implanted inside the body (lines 564–567). At lines 571 and 575, Dr. D isolates Mr Spencer's preference (you). The first time, line 571, points to the choice between PVAD BiVAD and HVAD BiVAD. The PVAD BiVAD requires less preparation and organization and, therefore, less time during which Mr Spencer can develop more arrhythmias. The second time (line 569) is the discussion about a possible ECMO procedure. In highlighting Mr Spencer's preference "you," Dr. D voices to Mr Spencer that his preferences are acknowledged. However, having defined the second "currently a *thou*ght" (line 574), Mr Spencer's rejection of a possible ECMO procedure is not yet accepted as the final decision by the doctor.

Dr. D, Dr. S, and CCU Nurse N in cogen have discussed their preoccupation with Mr Spencer not having yet grasped the nature of the potential bridge to a bridge (ECMO). Indeed, a few minutes earlier in the encounter (line 489), Mr Spencer confuses the ECMO procedure with open-heart surgeries. The healthcare professionals, in addition, discussed Mr Spencer's fear of futile interventions when in the hand of a doctor, Dr. S (and his surgical team), whom Mr Spencer just met.

Dr. D continues. He supports Dr. S's description, downsizing the ECMO implantation compared to BiVAD implantation and heart transplantation. He defines it as a catheter procedure (lines 577–579). Therefore, as Dr. S has done, he amends Mr Spencer's understanding of a three-stage procedure rather than two (BiVAD implantation with possible ECMO as a bridge to transplantation). By highlighting Mr Spencer's preferences first and then at lines 583 to 584 and 585 stating his opinion, Dr. D points to the role distribution. The patient has the right to make a final decision in consultation with the professional who needs to state their professional advice and discuss it with the patient and family. By doing so, Dr. D defines this process as a shared decision-making process. Dr. D expresses his assessment of accepting the possibility of ECMO implantation as "a very favorable decision" (line 584).

After Dr. D's words, the situation's intensity seems to have lost the turbulence generated by the ECMO team's sudden entry; however, as a coda, the loud sound of a beeper suddenly erupts. The ECMO team enters the conversation with Mr Spencer putting electrodes on his chest and side (lines 588–589). The defibrillator's mechanical voice speaks the automated words: *backup without signs of compression backup without signs of compression, bit bit bit* the heart monitor marks the accelerated heartbeats generated by a new v-tach episode.

Dr. D sighs loudly (line 590):

588	ECMO M2:	we are putting them as a backup now?
		backup without signs of compression
589		We are not planning to give you shock?
		backup without signs of compression
590	Dr. D:	(hhH)HHH ((deep loud sighs))
591	CCU Nurse N:	just putting them on
		bit bit bit bit bit bit bit bit bit
592	Dr. D:	(hhH)HHH share your thoughts anytime (hh)hh
		bit bit bit bit bit bit bit bit bit
593		I now want us to (.) work through this you know
594	Mr. Spencer:	I don't want (hh) ((as if about to cry))
595		stuff hanging out uh
		bit bit bit bit bit bit bit bit bit
596		except for an electrical cord or
		bit bit bit bit bit bit bit bit bit
597		that that's why that's acceptable
		bit bit bit bit bit bit bit bit bit
598		it would let me go home (0.4) for a while
		bit bit bit bit bit bit bit bit bit
599	Dr. D:	**yes**
		bit bit bit bit bit bit bit bit bit
600	Mr. Spencer:	till we had a transplant and have a somewhat normal **lif**e=
		bit bit bit bit bit bit bit bit bit

601   Dr. D: =the HVAD BiVAD *absolutely*=
                         bit bit bit   bit bit bit   bit bit bit

bit bit bit bit bit bit bit bit bit the three beats per second sound of
ventricular tachycardia (v-tach) now is ongoing and clearly audible via
the audio signal of the heart rhythm motor. The situation can turn into
an emergency if the v-tach does not quickly dissipate as it did before.
Dr. D's sighs (lines 590 and 592) are deep, conveying the gravity of what
is happening. He asks Mr Spencer to share his thoughts, "I now want us to
(.) work through this you know" (line 593) as he had shared in cogen "to
deliver the patient to the surgical team in a meaningful way that is with an
authentic decision made." Together they review the decisions in place once
again: Mr Spencer does not want to see the pumps pumping his blood outside
his body; the electrical cord will connect the pumps inside his body to the
batteries and computers (lines 595–596). He wants to be able to go home
(line 598) and recover there with a somewhat normal life (line 600). Dr. D
immediately translates Mr Spencer's decision into the available choice: the
HVAD BiVAD, emphasizing they agree (*yes*, line 599; *absolutely*, line 601).

602 Mr Spencer: =I've been in the hospital [for
                   bit bit bit   bit bit bit   bit bit bit
603 Dr. S: [you know
                   DU::::M   DU:::::M   DU::::M ((alarm of displaced electrodes))
                   bit bit bit   bit bit bit   bit bit bit
604 Dr. D: that [would be the goal

605 Dr. S: [you know the ECMO
                   bit bit bit   bit bit bit   bit bit bit
606   the ECMO circuit is uh
                   bit bit bit   bit bit bit   bit bit bit
607   very akin to what you had with the uhm impella device?
                   bit bit bit   bit bit bit   bit bit bit
608   it has sort of a=
                   bit bit bit   bit bit bit   bit bit bit
609 Dr. D: =that's the same it's very similar [so that's why
610 Dr. S: [it's a it's a
                   bit bit bit   bit bit bit   bit bit bit

611   it's a bigger tu:be it has you'll actually
                   bit bit bit   bit bit bit   bit bit bit

612   if you were conscious
                   bit bit bit   bit bit bit   bit bit bit

613   you'll actually see the blood (.) but uh
bit bit bit   bit bit bit   bit bit bit

614   We take the sickest patients u:h
bit bit bit   bit bit bit   bit bit bit

615   *to* the point where they can be candidates for (.) everything else
bit bit bit   bit bit bit   bit bit bit

Dr. S joins Dr. D and Mr Spencer. Dr. S intervenes (line 603), overlapping first with Mr Spencer (lines 603) and then with Dr. D (line 605) to describe the ECMO as well as the Impella device[3] (lines 606–608), something that Mr Spencer had when he was rushed to the emergency room weeks prior. Yes, that is very similar; Dr. D tries to regain space (line 609), but Dr. S, again as if in a relay race, does not relinquish the baton he just acquired (line 605), instead he continues the description of the ECMO device. However, Mr Spencer is not interested in what the device is. He is interested in how the machine impacts his short- and long-term life:

616   Mr. Spencer: i'm laying flat on my back the whole time?
617   Dr. S: you cannot walk with them
618   you're absolutely right
619   you lay on your back uhm

Dr. S starts answering Mr Spencer's question; however, *bit bit bit bit bit bit bit bit bit,* the v-tach does not stop. The urgent situation turns into an emergency.

620   Dr. S: MY FEELING is [that
621   Dr. D: [but it's [only also for a very few [days that
622   Dr. S: [yes   [a day or two
623   Dr. D   that you know
624   this is not a (0.4) living on the VA-ECMO
625   Dr. S: no:
626   Dr. D: this [is a (.) an *acute* support to
627   Dr. S: [no no right
628   Dr. D: a (.) decision making (.) [to do the uhm
629   Dr. S: [at most it's two to [three days

---

[3]The Impella is a device inserted through the arteries (percutaneously) rather than through "open heart surgery" that works similarly to a VAD helping the heart ventricle(s) pumping blood through the body. It is formally a *short-term* VAD.

```
630   Dr. D:                                        [a long term
631              [assist pump
632   Dr. S:     [while we get your
633   Dr. D:     [a-few-days
634   Dr. S:     [your situation [clarified and
635   Dr. D:                     [no-more-than that
636   Dr. S:     make sure your brain
637              is everything is okay after you went on it and
638              then and then
639              we would go but it's not a long term uh=
```

FRONTSTAGE		BACKSTAGE	
640 Dr D:	= it's very similar conceptually to the uhm	Dr S :	*(turns to talks to ECMO team and*
641	impella that you had in [outside hospital]		*AdHF Fellow))*
642	very very similar on the you know		*((not audible))*
643	it's a *short* *te*rm support until a emh		or redline him to the OR
644	next step is taken for a few days		do we have everything in place for
645			the VA:D
646 Dr D:	Yea::h		
647		AdHF F	I mean it would be okay

```
648 Dr S:   Do we have all the administrative stuff in place?
649 Dr D:   Yes yes that's in place
```

Both Dr. D and Dr. S immediately act as they are used to in their respective practices, taking charge in an emergency. Their overlaps show their moves. Dr. S suspends answering Mr Spencer's question and, with a loud voice, as shifting into a higher gear, moves fast into convincing Mr Spencer of the benefit of the ECMO. Dr. D does the same. The apparent competition for the lead fast resolves in organized teamwork: Dr. D talks to Mr Spencer and his family in frontstage to and Dr. S organizes the plan backstage. This is a boundary space, where a sudden change of a situation, from an urgency to an emergency, requires multiple rapid adjustments.

```
650              du:::m du::::m du::::m du:::m du::::m du::::m du:::m du:::m du:::m du::::m du:::m du:::m du::::m
                 du:::m du:::m
651   ECMO:      I don't want to leave him in this?
652              We want want to ATP him out of it
653   CCU Nurse: Would you like it in V1
                 BE::: BE:::: BE::::
                 bit bit bit    bit bit bit    bit bit bit

654   Mr. Spencer: I haven't changed my mind

                 bit bit bit    bit bit bit    bit bit bit
```

655	ECMO:	Okay starting ATP guys

bit bit bit   du:m   bit bit bit   du:m   bit bit bit   du:m   bit bit bit   du:m   bit bit
du:m
DU:::M DU:::::M DU:::M DU:::M DU:::::M DU:::M DU:::M DU::::: M DU:::M
DU:::M DU:: DU:::::M DU:::M
Hu:r Hu:r Hu: Hu: Hu:
BE::: BE::: BE:::

656	Dr. D:	would you like a (.) moment with wife and dad without us being here
657	Mr. Spencer:	*Uhm (10.0) ((the rest of the team talk to ecmo team in the background))*
658		I don't I don't necessarily want you guys to leave
659		cause you're watching over my stability right now
660	Dr. D:	yes that's right
661	Mr. Spencer:	so what
662	Dr. D:	or uhm maybe we could just uh
663		can you both maybe also just share your thoughts *((addresses family))*
664		come here yeah *((team talking in the background))*
665		we can we can use this moment to to uh
666		respecting whatever you want to be done *((to Mr Spencer))*
667		to go through this right now
668		we have we have **all the** ti:me
669		you know?

The ECMO team charges the machine (line 650) to deliver electrical pacing impulses 10 bits/minute faster than Mr Spencer's v-tach heart rate (ATP, line 652). The emergency does not change Mr Spencer's mind about the ECMO procedure (line 654). The ECMO team proceeds to ATP (line 655). The v-tach stops.

Dr. D asks Mr Spencer if he would like a moment alone with his family (line 656). Mr Spencer's wife and brother have already voiced their hope that Mr Spencer would accept the ECMO procedure if necessary (lines 506 and 509). As Dr. D reflected in cogen, with his family members, Mr Spencer would feel in a safe and trusted existential space where he does not feel pressured by the actions of the AdHF team. But Mr Spencer is scared to be left without medical supervision, watching over his stability (lines 657–659). Dr. D repeats the invitation. However, this time, he directly addresses the family that had retreated from the bed during the ECMO team's work. Dr. D invites them to share their thoughts with the promise of respecting Mr Spencer's preferences and supporting him in a shared decision-making process; "we have **all the** time, you know?" (line 668) In cogen session, Dr. D comments:

> Dr. D: Listening to this sentence, "we have all the time," I feel myself in that situation, trying to create an atmosphere where Mr Spencer

feels in a space that is not rushed, not driven, not motivated by the fear of dying and the associated anxiety in the team; the urgency, the indicators, like the alarms and the behavior of people, talking about the illnesses as opposed to talking about it with him. So, I'm seeing myself actively creating a contra-punctual atmosphere; is like Johann Sebastian Bach's composition.

It is interesting to see myself working on this. Just take what we just listen to, those five sentences [lines 663–668]. The last one of these is "we have all the time" [line 668], which is absurd; we have no time because right now he is dying. The sentence before is "respecting whatever you want" [line 666], and the sentence before this one is to his father, brother, and his wife to stand by next to him. They were basically paralyzed and not interacting with him. So I'm trying to ease them into saying something to this patient who is at risk of dying right now. The sentence before this is "share your thoughts" [line 663]. It's the first of the five. I went backward. "Share your thoughts," and it is so important for me to listen to this; my voice is contra-punctual to everything else that's going on. It's the opposite of the high pitch of all the alarms and alarmed voices. I am trying to own the space with the patient that allows for some existential and spiritual connections and against the gradient of the emergency.

The Resident doctor participating in cogen responds to Dr. D:

R: I totally agree. In this moment, Dr. S and the ECMO team, like everyone else, are moving in one direction: start ECMO! Save the patient! Like: we don't have ANY time. Dr. D and the patient are taking a moment, a different direction. The sentence 'we have all the time' was so funny to me; my heart rate started speeding up; even just listening to the situation, I felt like there is no time! We have no time! Dr. D takes the power because he's making time as if there was time, 'we are creating time' based on the patient's values, dying versus getting a procedure against his will. You [Dr. D] are balancing that all. I think it speaks to how well you [Dr. D] understand the patient, you know, and I think also the patient signals to you that he understands how seriously ill he is, and you listen. A lot of docs would think that the patient doesn't get it, you know, because he is blocking a potentially lifesaving procedure. But Mr. Spencer understands. He says I don't think you should leave the room because you're watching over me because I'm unstable. So he signals to you that he gets it, you get it. And the patient has the power to stop [the procedure]. So both you and the patient are having the power in this moment because every other physician and nurse in that room are like, "Go! Go! Go!" preparing for that moment, and the patient is saying "I'm not sure yet." Saying 'we have all the time' honestly almost makes you laugh in a way because it's so . . . In a doctor-centered perspective, it's so crazy to say that because we don't have time. In the doctor's typical perception, it's like we have to save this person's life, and we don't have that much time. The way we cope with that stress is to do something, you know, and they're all moving towards that, and it takes a lot to stop that momentum, yeah, and create that space. So, it is in contrast to everyone else's pace in the room and also me as a listener, because even me as a listener, I'm like, oh my God, he's going to code right there if we don't start ECMO. I know listening to this, I, I can't imagine doing what you did in this moment because I still have, I just feel the adrenaline. I think that would be really hard to do in that moment for me. I think it's very impressive.

The discussion among the healthcare professionals in cogen points to two aspects. Attending doctors and those at different stages of training (e.g., Resident, Fellow) *highlight* the situation as relevant, pausing the recording to comment on this moment. They all *code* the situation as very urgent with the possibility of degenerating into an emergency. However, the emotional responses are different. While the Resident and the cardiology Fellow, feeling the adrenaline rising, are drawn into the room's emergency mood, the AdHF Attending, Dr. D, acts differently. The Resident describes Dr. D's counter-punctual move to the emergency mood as "stopping that momentum" that drew all, including the Resident, into an emergency mood.

Both the Resident and Fellow recognize Dr. D's capacity to make a counter-punctual move as a "very impressive" skill that helps the patient partake in a shared decision-making process. They also point out that it is a skill they did not master yet. Their assessment points to what is relevant for them to learn, to become the kind of doctor that helps the patient partake in a shared decision-making.

Affordances in Teamwork

Dr. D's advanced skills and his way of being a doctor are undoubtedly necessary to account for the counter-punctual move; however, they are not enough to accomplish it. Indeed, with a suddenly changing situation, from urgent to emergency at the onset of the ventricular tachycardia, the immediate "stress reaction," as the Resident reports, is to "do something!" Both the Attendings, Dr. D and Dr. S, immediately moved to take the lead in the fast pace of an emergency. However, a boundary space characterized by multiple rapid adjustments of the Attendings' apparent competition for the lead emerges (lines 620–639) and fast resolves into organized teamwork with coordinated actions and activities necessary to care for Mr Spencer. Specifically, Dr. D talks to Mr Spencer and his family in the frontstage, and Dr. S starts organizing the plan for surgery in the backstage (line 640–647). Within the larger background context of caring for Mr Spencer, the local organization of the two professionals' responses is organized according to the diversified *professional goals* and *anticipated actions*. Dr. D's goal, as he has expressed earlier, "is to deliver the patient to the surgical team in a meaningful way that is with an authentic decision made." Dr. S' goal is to consent Mr Spencer and prepare the surgery for a safe procedure with a successful outcome. The fast reorganization and division of backstage and frontstage activities show how well Dr. S and Dr. D know how to rely on each other and support their respective professional goals and needs, which combined provide the care Mr Spencer needs. Dr. S and Dr. D have worked closely together for the past years; with the shared background of caring for the patient, they continuously monitor each other's differential actions making sure they contribute to the complementary final goal of care.

This cooperation allows Dr. D to take a counter-punctual stream of actions that ensure that Mr Spencer can have a safe space to share his thoughts and prayer with his family in a decisive moment of his care. It is based on this that Dr. S, as he also discussed in the cogen, could, a few moments later, leave Mr Spencer's CCU room to come back after Mr Spencer and his family, under the supervision of Dr. D, had time to talk and pray together.

CHAPTER 8

CONCLUSION

We started our book at the end. In Chapter 1, we followed Dr. D's presentation at the Annual Heart Failure Symposium, more than one year after the encounters with Mr Spencer. There, Dr. D asks the audience to choose one of the two options:

If Mr Spencer would code now, who would:

Choice 1 — let him die peacefully in concordance with his expressed preferences, and who would

Choice 2 — let him pass out and become unconscious from the v-tach/v-fib, then turn to his wife — his surrogate decision-maker — standing next to him at the bedside and follow her advice to put Mr Spencer on Venoarterial Extracorporeal Membrane Oxygenation (VA-ECMO) as a short-term bridge to (Ventricular Assist Device [VAD]) and heart transplantation?

and then . . .

and then we left the scene. Now we return to it:

Upon concluding his case presentation, Dr. D invites heart transplant patients present in the Heart Failure Symposium Lecture Hall to join him on the podium. Four persons walk to the front, up the stairs to the podium, and sit at a long table. Dr. D addresses the first: "Would you care to comment"?

"[. . .] When that day comes for me, I don't want to go kicking and screaming

Our days are numbered, [. . .] It seemed like my days were up. [. . .]

How much time do we have? All the time you need [. . .] Dr. D and the team allowed me and my family to pray [. . .] I am glad I did!"

The symposium audience applauds, recognizing Mr Spencer.

A *few months later*, in his lecture for the Residents in the CCU conference room, Dr. D describes: "[. . .] and after that vote was cast at the Heart Failure Symposium Lecture Hall, I asked Mr. Spencer to come to the podium." Like the audience's applause at the symposium, a liberating laughter surges from the Residents.

Dr. D continues:

> I had not disclosed his presence to the Heart Failure Symposium attendees. I asked him to come up and share his thoughts. So now, obviously, you are missing something in between, right?

The Residents giggle.

Dr. D: And so, what happened was, fortunately, he did not code. So, fortunately, it didn't lead to this situation that is so challenging. What happened was what I started talking about already; there was the sentence intermingled into this situation. I think we're scaring him, said someone. And then I transformed this into I think we're scaring you.

And that transformed into Dr. S saying maybe we should give you some time[1] with your loved ones without us being here. And then the patient says the sentence: Yes, but you're watching over my life, and I don't know if I have the time, and then, in that moment, I'm saying a sentence that comes out of me: we have all the time. And I think then comes a decision ... Mr. Spencer requests CCU nurse N and me to stay in the room while everyone else is leaving, and then it takes about twenty minutes where he starts praying, his wife starts praying with him, and the parents start praying with him. And twenty or so minutes later, he turns to me and asks: Dr. D, so tell me again, what is this VA-ECMO about exactly? And then I explain again that if necessary, next twenty-four hours, while we're waiting for the HVAD-BiVAD to arrive, that we will have you in VA-ECMO standby. Then we put the HVAD-BiVAD in and then the transplant, and then he says, well, if it's just for that short period of time, I think I can do it. And then Dr. S comes back in, and Mr. Spencer says to me, if you, Dr. D, could please explain what we just discussed to

---

[1] It is interesting to note that in Dr. D's narrative, it is not him but Dr. S who said, "maybe we should give you some time with your loved ones without us being here." We interpret this not simply as a vague memory of what happened, but as Dr. D having a sense of belonging to a team working together and allowing the other member of the team to build on each other to care for Mr Spencer.

Dr. S, so I have this certainty that we're all on the same page. And I explained that. And that includes what was not contentious at all:

Should I have a stroke? I want to be let go.
Should I be on dialysis? I want to be let go.

No one questioned that at all. So, after we repeat this all together, Mr. Spencer says, 'yeah, okay, now I'm ready to go for this.

Becoming a Team

From December 24 to January 1, Mr Spencer, his family, and the Advanced Heart Failure (AdHF) team have confronted numerous uncertainties together. We showed how Dr. D *framed for and with* Mr Spencer these uncertainties, centering them around Mr Spencer's expectations and existential queries. Dr. D not only attended to Mr Spencer's thinking or his intellectual understanding of options and procedures but *cared* for Mr Spencer (Raia, 2018, 2020b) as a person who is existentially shaken by the very real possibility of losing his heart, losing his way of life and facing death. In Chapter 3, e.g., Dr. D's acts of care are accomplished by the doctor's talk punctuated by silences and repetitions. His talk creates a space in which Mr Spencer's doubts about new uncertainties and complex options can emerge; a space where the uncertainties can be discussed, can be framed for and with Mr Spencer when Mr Spencer is prepared to do so (e.g., December 29, lines 66–68). Dr. D's acts of care are accomplished as relational ability to attend to the interactions between Mr Spencer and other professionals, e.g., in Chapter 4, with trainee novices of the AdHF practice, and with other professionals, such as the ECMO team in Chapter 7.

On January 1, Dr. D, Mr Spencer, and his family need to navigate new uncertainties. Mr Spencer meets his surgeon for the first time on a day in which Mr Spencer fears that, due to the "weekend effect, not "the best team" is available" (see Chapter 6, January 1, lines 122–127). Mr Spencer possibly needs an emergency bridge to a bridge to transplantation (ECMO) while continuing to be fearful of what can be done to him in high-tech medicine. Indeed, a few minutes later in the encounter (not reported here), Mr Spencer tells his family: "if I authorize everything, everything could be done for hours. They could open up my chest and do everything for a long period of time; we heard how long that code blue might get enacted; that's scarier than dying to me."

During the escalation from urgency to emergency, Dr. D, in collaboration with the other members of the AdHF team, creates again a space that Mr Spencer needs where there is "all the time" for Mr Spencer.

Mr Spencer and Mrs Spencer later recount.

> Mr Spencer: Dr. S made his case that he needed the option of an external pump during the surgery. If it became necessary, a pump accessing an artery in my leg could keep my body's blood circulation flowing throughout the surgery. Dr. D was keeping everyone calm and patient, both inside the room and apparently outside in the hall as well. I asked if we could have some time to pray. "How much time do we have to make a decision?" I asked. "All the time you need." he calmly replied. His serenity was part of what kept me from perceiving just how dire things had become. Polite, patient, and respectful, Dr. D stayed with us while we prayed around the room for about twenty minutes. [wife's name], [son's and daughter's names], and my dad were all there. As we spoke after praying, they all expressed their wish for me to give the okay. It seemed ghoulish and a desperate grasping to hold on to a life that God seemed to be steadily removing me from, but I agreed.

> Mrs Spencer: He [Mr. Spencer] didn't want the mechanical heart support [ECMO] and the family all decided to pray around him. Dr. D put his hand on [Mr. Spencer]'s arm and he stood there with us and he just waited for us to have that time together praying. His presence was just there the whole time. Very, very supportive. And I think that the decision had a lot to do with.

In concluding Chapter 7, we discussed the power of teamwork in affording Dr. D's counter-punctual move. However, there is more to it. Through a process of *framing for and with the Other*, Dr. D, Mr Spencer, and his family also have been building trustful relations allowing Dr. D to take a counter-punctual stream of actions ensuring that Mr Spencer has a safe space to share his thoughts and pray. Mr Spencer, his family, CCU Nurse N, Dr. D, and the other multidisciplinary AdHF members, including Dr. S, who Mr Spencer meet last, have become a team.

Learning to Care for the Other

Interpreted within the Relational Ontology framework (Raia, 2018, 2020; forthcoming), when Dr. D creates a space for Mr Spencer and his family to pray and, partaking in it as a professional, he identifies Mr Spencer's spiritual life as salient for all. Mr Spencer is a religious and spiritual man. Praying is a part of his life as an existential past modulating his sensibility to attune to what is relevant to him and a future sense of possibilities of being himself so that Mr Spencer can inhabit a meaningful and shared present with the physician to face the decision to accept an ECMO.

As Raia and Deng (2015b) discuss, it requires a long-term process of attunement to the Other developing during the daily meetings as a recursive process. Indeed, it is made possible based on the iteration aspect of the AdHF encounters. It is not a linear process of adding new information and new knowledge, but a process of learning to care for this person. Learning how to care for Mr Spencer. While, in the long-term, attunement to the Other develops, Dr. D responds also to the specific situation. A short-term moment-to-moment synchronization with the Other and to the dynamic situation of the encounter. As Dr. D recounts in cogen:

> Dr. D: "It comes out of the moment. I found it very interesting that I said the sentence standing next to him [Mr. Spencer] and — you've seen me with patients — I'm saying we have all the time in the context of Dip Dip Dip Dip and have to put an a-line in, have to anti-tachycardia pace (ATP) him out of it. You know, it's clearly a background that doesn't feel like a very meditative time to — in this situation of his — pray, which enables him to come to a decision." Dr. D continues sharing with the cogen research team his interaction with the residents during the resident lecture, "Now, that links into another question that you've been asking and everybody wanted to know, is he really present? Is he really functional? Can he really make decisions? Now, on the surface, clearly. Absolutely. Yes. But I have to conclude that he hadn't really processed it, processed in the sense: actually, that's me. That is in that situation. And it's undetectable on the surface because it sounds all, sentence structure, semantics, you know, everything looks intact. No reason to doubt his decision-making capacity. But it wasn't processed.

I realize this, not even when he said, what's VA-ECMO all about? But when in the co-gen research meetings actually, because it's such an interesting moment, what actually does it make possible for a person to make a decision since we're not Volkswagens with a motor exchange, but persons, you know, and it's related to *me as a person* to make the decision. That's the challenge. How do I make decisions? Apparently that's one of the conclusions actually, for me as a person to make a decision, I need to have my basic human right of personhood respected, whatever that means. In order to do so, apparently, the health care professional needs to be available as a person to care for me as a person, whatever that means again in that moment."

I realized when I say we have all the time, it was more on that level that I was, I think, available for him to say, okey, I want to pray. So, there's something in this care concept that we, I think, need as a framework of our practice that then makes everything that high-tech medicine has to offer meaningful.

Dr. D reports this reflection also in his lecture to the Residents and adds:

"I think it's very important that everybody develops a practice framework with a value system where you anticipate that at 1:00 a clock in the morning you're here and the Attendings are at home nicely asleep, you have to make decisions, utilize your own practice framework and be prepared that even 152 year old practitioners may not, although they are grey-haired, be necessarily more wise in their decision making framework of values. So you have your own values, take the stand, take the courage and argue whatever that is. And it might be at times conflictual. That's okay. And that comes out of a concept of care for the patients."

What Happened to Mr Spencer?

We understand that some may be curious to know what happened to Mr Spencer between the encounter on January 1 and his appearance at the symposium, as the Resident were.

We follow Dr. D's narrative as he recounts what happened to the Residents during his lecture in the CCU conference room.

Dr. D: "What happens next? We put Mr Spencer in the CTICU. He spends the night to January 2. Nothing happens. He does not need the ECMO. And on Saturday, January 2, he is implanted the HVAD-Biventricular Assist Device (BiVAD), our first Heartware-Right Ventricular Assist Device (RVAD), and Dr. S does it really well. And on Sunday, January 3, Mr. Spencer is extubated and is sitting in the chair. On Monday morning, January 4, he's walking in the CTICU, and everyone applauds. On Friday, January 8, in the Heart Transplant Selection Committee meeting, since he's doing so well, we activate him on the waiting list. And on Saturday, January 9, I received a phone call — one of my AdHF Attending colleagues is on call. I receive a phone call from him because I was taking care of Mr. Spencer during the last weeks, it is a Public Health Service (PHS) increased risk[2] organ, and we haven't even started consenting him for Public Health Service Increased Risk (PHS-IR) organs, so he has an organ offer, and over the phone, we have a 15 minute conversation where he says, okay, I'm going to go for that. So he has transplantation on January 9, on January 23 he's discharged, and in July he returns to work as his junior high school's principal. And then, in September, he starts teaching the seventh graders his new HVAD-BiVAD equipment that he had been using. So he takes all these artifacts home to make it part of health education."

The trustful relations established in this newly configured team are recognized by the others as essential. Indeed, when a heart offer is received for Mr Spencer, the AdHF cardiologist, who is the Attending on-call that week, asks Dr. D to call Mr Spencer to tell him about the offer and discuss with him what is an organ designated "Public Health Service Increased Risk."

---

[2]Public Health Service Increased Risk identifies donors who, based on life styles or experiences, are at increased risk of transmitting hepatitis B, C, and human immunodeficiency virus. In 2007, the Organ Procurement and Transplantation Network (OPTN) started requiring documentation of patients informed consent for the acceptance of such organs (Seem *et al.*, 2013). With the PHS IR label associated with low utilization with loss of hundreds of organs per year (Volk *et al.*, 2017), with increased capacity to detect donor issues and disease transmission possibilities along with a more diffuse process of shared decision-making to understand the minimal risk associated with the use of PHS-IR organs (Moayedi *et al.*, 2018); in 2021, new guidelines (UNOS, 2021) were issued that requires the delivery of information to patient and family about the risk rather than specific, separate informed consent.

Our Approach to Concluding This Book

We think that a reflection of what is learned or discovered by the practitioners during our work through all the stages of our research model is the best conclusion for this book. We proceed by discussing the recurring aspects of every encounter and multi-encounter episode themes that the Attendings have discussed and Dr. D, in particular, has reflected upon during our collaborative work. We hope to provide important training/teaching/education modules and themes, for the medical practitioners. We will reflect on these Relational Medicine themes in the context of the widely adopted fellowship development milestones developed by the United States Accreditation Council for Graduate Medical Education (ACGME) that were originally published in 2014. Indeed, Graduate Medical Education Programs (Residency and Fellowship) are currently expected to implement these ACGME Milestones for the training and assessment of trainees' competence in medical procedures and patient care. The original model of skill acquisition upon which the milestones were developed was based on the phenomenological studies of chess players, air force pilots, and army tank drivers and commanders (Dreyfus & Dreyfus, 1988). As phenomenological studies, the analyses are grounded in the specific experiences of the participant trainers and trainees, the affordances and solicitations to which they respond, what becomes salient in their interactions with tools, equipment, and interlocutors. In the process of adaptation of the Dreyfus model in graduate medical education, various competencies were defined a priori for the different medical disciplines and related specialties by expert ACGME subcommittees. Each of those competencies were further divided along five skill levels (levels 1–5) each representing a stage of competency level in Dreyfus's model, with the highest level as the target skill level for trainees at the completion of training.

In their presentation of the Milestones project, Batalden *et al.* (2002) identified a substantial challenge in the appropriate adaptation and implementation as assessment tool of the ACGME Milestones to each professional medical discipline. Specifically, they reported that in each original category of skill acquisition well-meaning but too abstract additional process specifications were added to target the professional preparation process, resulting in an exponential increase in the number of "musts" and "shoulds" that disjoined these well-reasoned process prescriptions from their application in daily healthcare practice. As Batalden *et al.* (2002) argue: "Further, they have inadvertently contributed to a preoccupation on matters away from the 'core' of physician specialist preparation. Departing program directors with short terms of duty have shared their frustrations of trying to link these well-meaning process prescriptions to daily work in today's health care as a major contributor to their short tenure" (p. 110).

In this chapter, we intend, starting from the abstract training goals and the specific practice of training in patient care, to make suggestions how — based on our "Relational Ontology" research method described in Chapter 2 and applied to the situation of Mr Spencer in Chapters 3 to 7 — we may facilitate understanding of (1) specific practices and (2) training concepts that are transferable to other medical practice training settings. To dive into the dilemma of what the well-intended but too abstract specification of the ACGME Cardiovascular Disease Milestones (Second Revision, December 2020) looks like and how our approach may help get out of the dilemma, we present our interpretation of the Level 4/5 performance in the situation of taking care of Mr Spencer.

Let us start at the beginning of our case analysis of Mr Spencer in Chapter 1: Dr. D presents Mr Spencer's case at the May 6 Heart Failure Symposium and the December 21 Resident lecture. We interpret this act of Dr. D as Level 5 practice, i.e., he "Disseminates knowledge of challenging presentations and uncommon disorders" (Medical Knowledge 2: Critical Thinking for Diagnosis and Therapy, ACGME Cardiovascular Disease Milestones, Second Revision, December 2020) and he "Develops initiatives to educate others to critically appraise and apply evidence for complex patients and/or participates in the development of guidelines" (Practice-Based Learning and Improvement 1: Evidence-based and Informed Practice, ACGME Cardiovascular Disease Milestones, Second Revision, December 2020).

Let us now continue with a detailed account of Dr. D's care for Mr Spencer, starting from the crisis moment and the crisis-turning sentence "We have all the time" (Chapter 7). While reviewing the encounter episodes with Mr Spencer from December 29 to January 1, we will touch upon the various themes summarized below and will interpret them in the context of the ACGME milestones.

Exploring third options by focusing on moment-to-moment interactions

A sentence such as "We have all the time" cannot be understood, practiced, taught, and learned in isolation, as a context-free isolated Relational*Act*. Rather, it has to be interpreted in the situational context.

I, Dr. D, see myself as part of a multidisciplinary team. I know and trust my team members to take care — in this very moment — of the urgent "clock time" issues on backstage. This trust into the team and teamwork allows me to fully immerse myself into the patient's existential perspective. This move allows me to attune (Raia & Deng, 2015b) to what gives birth to the Relational*Act* (*notabene:* not reductionist speech act) "We have all the time."

Another prerequisite — in addition to trusting the team — is the building of a safe space and trusting relationship with Mr Spencer over the preceding days in the process of framing the options (see Chapter 2). The creation of a safe space that allows for deep listening, meaningful silences, and appreciation of the healthcare professional's own mortality culminates in the professional vision of presentness, i.e., being and acting in the "here and now" in the multi-adic encounter with patient and family. This mindset then allows the healthcare professional to say sentences such as "We have all the time" (Chapter 7).

Initiating relationalact-encounters openly and inclusively

This safe space trusting relationship is initiated in a proactive way, as Dr. D states in cogen: "My experience tells me to be proactive in the very first meeting with patient and family. There are three things that I always do: first, I give them my business card so they can get in touch with me anytime, including calling my cellphone. Second, I sit down to talk with the patient and family. Third, I outline the scenarios . . ." (Chapter 3).

Creating safe spaces

How do we, as healthcare professionals, know that we have been successful in building a safe space in an encounter with a specific patient? We have to interpret the other person's — the patient's — feedback, as, e.g., Mr Spencer describes in his account: "Dr. D proved to be an incredibly personal and tuned-in doctor. From the first introduction he remembered all my family members' names. He sincerely wanted to hear our concerns and apprehensions, took the time to answer all our questions, and always kept us well informed with each new development and options to be considered. Only when we had nothing more to ask would he start to leave, with a warm smile, and the words, 'to be continued.' With such a rare disease, and so many unknowns, here was a man who could speak knowledgeably and reassuringly about my diagnosis and possible approaches. What a blessing from God." (Chapter 3).

Framing evidence-based options

From our Relational Medicine perspective, the creation of a safe space is the initial goal of highest priority during every encounter. It creates the basis for presenting and framing the different treatment options as guiding perspective for all future encounters, as Dr. D states: "I usually say 'just for the sake of completeness, it's worth talking about all the options that could theoretically come up." Most of them feel very theoretical kind of general picture, because they are not affecting the patient right now. But at the same time, talking about the potential scenarios in AdHF, one of which will eventually become the actual one, becomes part of the overall plan from the get go. So, to later on come back to our first discussion is much more straightforward and feels much better than to say, at a later stage, when things are getting into a downward spiral in a crisis mode: "by the way, we now have to talk about another option' that a patient never heard of before" (Chapter 3). By doing so, not only does the **patient** experience the continuity in the care process, but so does the **healthcare professional**.

Acknowledging uncertainty

From the Relational Medicine practitioner's professional vision perspective, it seems necessary to be prepared to be comfortable with uncertainty and proactively acknowledge the various domains of uncertainty. Doing so, will facilitate meaningful decision-making by the patient, e.g., in Dr. D's statement "from that time point on to transplantation is not (1.0) an hour period, it's not (.) a day period, it's not necessarily a week period, it's not necessarily a month period" (Chapter 3). Neglecting to do so, creates potentially hazardous misconceptions for the patient. It is interesting to note that Dr. D's appreciation of uncertainty (see Chapter 2) was perceived by Mr Spencer as "reassuring" (Chapter 3).

Availing oneself by listening deeply for questions and explanations

Framing the options and their associated uncertainties creates an invitation of potential patient and caregiver/family questions. Having entered this existential space, "deep" listening is required to invite the patient to develop an understanding what choosing a specific option means in her or his life, what "makes sense." Phrases such as "that's a very good question" (Chapter 3) are conducive to creating a "deep" listening atmosphere in the safe space.

Allowing silences

As important as "deep" listening are silences that allow for "sinking in" time of insights in the safe space, as described in the scene "After a silence that did elicit neither further elaboration nor other thoughts or information from Mr. Spencer, Dr. D with "okay" (line 22), marking the beginning of a new activity (Beach, 1993, 1995), zooms in on the relevant event since their last visit the day prior, "how was your night?" (Chapter 5).

Appreciating own mortality

Another essential facet of the safe space RelationalAct encounter is the appreciation by the healthcare professional of their own mortality as a necessary condition for the "deep" listening process and the silences. I (Dr. D) have come to use the scripted phase "cause honestly it's unlikely that thousand years from now we'll be standing in this room? (.) and discussing things (1.3) although it's not completely predictable? (1.5)" (Chapter 5).

Embedding clock time in existential time

Allowing existentially important activities for the patient and their loved ones such as meditation or praying to integrate the past/memories and future projections allows Mr Spencer to be present in the existential time safe space of "here and now" to make clock time life and death decisions.

This concept is explicated in Chapter 5: how to project a person into future possibilities of being *this person* after having grounded the person in a common existential past is crucial in caring for the Other. Projecting Mr Spencer into imagining the action he can take toward recovery is a big step into Mr Spencer's existential future and Chapter 6: "the doctor creates a temporal horizon" (Raia, 2020): he first grounds Mr Spencer in a common existential past, which is quite recent in terms of clock time, just a few days, but existentially very significant as Mr Spencer's life has been changing dramatically. Dr. D calls upon their common existential past by pointing to their critical discussions preparing for these changes in Mr Spencer's life a few days prior (lines 296–297). Then, Dr. D projects Mr Spencer into future possibilities of being with his wife. Grounding Mr Spencer in a common past and projecting him into future possibility of being himself, Dr. D can reframe the question and current understanding of the "big picture."

Explicating role distributions

When during the Relational*Act* encounter decision-making is approaching, I (Dr. D) have come to appreciate the proactive statement that in the safe space "there's a certain role distribution um that I feel us white coats make recommendations and the boss makes decisions" (Chapter 5).

Sharing decision-making

In the Relational Medicine framework, we are sharing decision-making in the sense of a collaborative decision-making, conceptualized as an ongoing multi-adic process with continuous negotiations, e.g., as in "that would be an important in my opinion a very favorable decision to make . . ." (Chapter 7).

Applying caring power

In these negotiations, healthcare professionals use different techniques including soft power as exemplified in """viruses, bacteria, and fungi" having a happy life" (Chapter 3).

Embracing inclusive "we" ness

The shared/collaborative decision-making process benefits — from the Relational Medicine perspective — from an as-inclusive-as-possible use of the concept of "we" such as discussed in "After having reported about the team discussion, Dr. D and the Fellows attended (line 1–3), Dr. D uses the pronoun "we" in an ambiguous way (lines 17–20): "that we (the team), as we (you and I) said yesterday hum are uhm observing since you came here and we (can point to exclusive or inclusive) started the therapy." English does not differentiate formally between exclusive and inclusive we. The lack of semantic distinction can point to a "we" used to include the patient, to mean you and I, or you, me and the team or we humans or to exclude the patient, to mean we the team (Skelton *et al.*, 2002). With a return to the use of unspecified subjects (line 21), the third we (line 20) would be expected to be inclusive." (Chapter 3).

Fostering teamwork

This inclusive "we" ness invites various team members, patient and family/caregiver into the Relational*Act* safe space for the ongoing shared/collaborative decision-making process, as Dr. D explains in cogen session: "Dr. D, inviting Dr. C to partake in the discussion of Mr. Spencer's care has four main outcomes: the first and most obvious is for Dr. D and the team to share their thoughts about Mr. Spencer's condition and treatment with another expert. The second is creating a team teaching environment, in which everybody could participate in learning also from experts' discussion. The third is communicating to the patient and the family, to whom Dr. D will report the discussion, that the team has looked at all the different options and possibilities in light of current scientific data so that there was no doubt on the part of the patient and the family that all that was possible was done. The fourth is to maintain a culture of team work, dismantling or preventing the formation of a sense that, with time and developed expertise, a doctor acquires all the necessary knowledge. To learn that the ethics of caring for people requires, as Dr. D put it, "to jump over one's own kind of shadows, our medical egos." (Chapter 5).

Attuning to multiparty conversation

Fostering team work and an inclusive concept of "we" requires a continuous process of attuning to a multiparty conversation, such as witnessed in "Dr. D accomplishes two critical goals. He welcomes the brother indicating that he knows about how vital the brother's contribution has been. He reestablishes

Mr. Spencer as the addressee and a speaker. Specifically, Dr. D engages in three subsequent actions: first, he builds on Mr. Spencer's brother's story about talking to Ms. Moose (lines 42–67, omitted). He acknowledges how helpful it is to have the opportunity to see how others have gone through similar medical and existential issues, and, in doing so, addresses Mr. Spencer directly (you, line 76). With this move, Mr. Spencer is again the primary addressee and speaker in the multi-party conversation, adverting the possibility of becoming an object about whom participants talk" (Chapter 5).

Observing the frontstage–backstage settings

In this multiparty conversation, it is essential that the healthcare professional team members develop an expert sensibility for backstage/frontstage appropriateness, such as expertly displayed by CCU Nurse N in: "his vEry devoted brother: who keeps a vE:ry close eye on him" (Chapter 5).

Noticing in multiactivity coexisting existential spaces

In this multiparty and multiactivity space, the healthcare professional's sensibility to distinguishing the patient care space from, e.g., the training space is essential, such as discussed in: "so ventricular assist device ((turns to the Fellows)) thanks for mentioning that specifically" (Chapter 4).

Operating transformations

An important expert tool is the reassignment of meaning/interpretation of an event/decision made by the patient: "Dr. S does not contradict Mr. Spencer, Mr. Spencer is right ("you're right there's not," line 135) people are not fresh at two o'clock in the morning (I would not like to go at two in the morning, line 137). Dr. S takes what is right in Mr Spencer's understanding and reframes it for him; the surgeon operates a transformation from "not the best team" into "they are not a special team" (Chapter 6).

Repairing communication acts

An important integration function in the Relational Medicine framework is the ability to repair prior RelationalActs, such as Dr. D demonstrates in "let's assume there is stability." Dr. D repairs the sentence (line 426) with "which uh may not be the case" (line 428) and treads carefully (Chapter 7).

Owning one's professional vision

Putting all these Relational Medicine Milestone themes to work provides a glimpse into and an invitation for participation in our Relational Medicine professional vision, based on the Relational Ontology framework (Raia, 2018, 2020) which itself is built on the shoulder of giants: In his seminal paper, professional vision, C. Goodwin (1994) demonstrates that the perceptions and understanding of events "are not idiosyncratic phenomena restricted to individuals but shared frameworks, domains of professional competence. [. . .] Socially organized ways of seeing and understanding events are answerable to the distinctive interests of a particular social group making up the work environment of a scientific discipline" (Chapter 7).

REFERENCES

ACGME (2020). ACGME program requirements for graduate medical education in advanced heart failure and transplant cardiology. https://www.acgme.org/globalassets/PFAssets/ProgramRequirements/159_AdvancedHeartFailureTransplantCardiology_2020.pdf?ver=2020-02-14-153940-843&ver=2020-02-14-153940-843

Alasuutari, P. (2018). Authority as epistemic capital. *Journal of Political Power, 11*(2), 165–190. https://doi.org/10.1080/2158379X.2018.1468151

Alby, F., Zucchermaglio, C., & Baruzzo, M. (2015). Diagnostic decision making in oncology: Creating shared knowledge and managing complexity. *Mind, Culture, and Activity, 22*(1), 4–22. https://doi.org/10.1080/10749039.2014.981642

Allen, L. A., McIlvennan, C. K., Thompson, J. S., Dunlay, S. M., LaRue, S. J., Lewis, E. F., Patel, C. B., Blue, L., Fairclough, D. L., Leister, E. C., Glasgow, R. E., Cleveland, J. C., Phillips, C., Baldridge, V., Walsh, M. N., & Matlock, D. D. (2018). Effectiveness of an intervention supporting shared decision making for destination therapy left ventricular assist device: The DECIDE-LVAD randomized clinical trial. *JAMA Internal Medicine, 178*(4), 520. https://doi.org/10.1001/jamainternmed.2017.8713

Allen, L. A., Stevenson, L. W., Grady, K. L., Goldstein, N. E., Matlock, D. D., Arnold, R. M., Cook, N. R., Felker, G. M., Francis, G. S., Hauptman, P. J., Havranek, E. P., Krumholz, H. M., Mancini, D., Riegel, B., & Spertus, J. A. (2012). Decision making in advanced heart failure: A scientific statement from the American heart association. *Circulation, 15*, 1928–1952.

Allman, R. M. (1985). Physician tolerance for uncertainty: Use of liver-spleen scans to detect metastases. *JAMA, 254*(2), 246. https://doi.org/10.1001/jama.1985.03360020078028

Armstrong, K. (2018). If you can't beat it, join it: Uncertainty and trust in medicine. *Annals of Internal Medicine, 168*(11), 818–819. https://doi.org/10.7326/M18-0445

Atkinson, P., & Heath, C. (1981). *Medical work: Realities and routines*. Gower.

Attali, J. (1985). *Noise: The political economy of music*. Manchester University Press.

Auer, P., Auer, P. L., Couper-Kuhlen, E., & Müller, F. (1999). *Language in time: The rhythm and Tempo of spoken interaction*. Oxford University Press.

Austin, J. L. (1965). *How to do things with words the William James lectures delivered at Harvard University in 1955*. Oxford University Press.

Babrow, A. S., Kasch, C. R., & Ford, L. A. (1998). The many meanings of uncertainty in illness: Toward a systematic accounting. *Health Communication, 10*(1), 1–23. https://doi.org/10.1207/s15327027hc1001_1

Bakhtin, M. (1981). *The dialogic imagination: Four essays* (M. Holquist, Ed.; C. Emerson & M. Holquist, Trans.). University of Texas Press.

Batalden, P., Leach, D., Swing, S., Dreyfus, H., & Dreyfus, S. (2002). General competencies and accreditation in graduate medical education. *Health Affairs, 21*(5), 103–111. https://doi.org/10.1377/hlthaff.21.5.103

Bateson, G. (1972). *Steps to an Ecology of Mind.* Ballantine Books.

Baum, F., MacDougall, C., & Smith, D. (2006). Participatory action research. *Journal of Epidemiology and Community Health, 60*(10), 854–857. https://doi.org/10.1136/jech.2004.028662

Beach, W. A. (1993). Transitional regularities for 'casual' "Okay" usages. *Journal of Pragmatics, 19*(4), 325–352. https://doi.org/10.1016/0378-2166(93)90092-4

Beach, W. A. (1995). Preserving and constraining options: Okays and official priorities in medical interviews. In *The Talk of the Clinic: Explorations in the Analysis of Medical and Therapeutic Discourse.* Erlbaum.

Beach, W. A. (2009). *A natural history of family cancer: Interactional resources for managing illness.* Hampton Press.

Beach, W. A. (2014). Managing hopeful moments: Initiating and responding to delicate concerns about illness and health. In *The Routledge Handbook of Language and Health Communication, 2014.* (pp. 459–476, 459–476). https://dialnet.unirioja.es/servlet/articulo?codigo$=$5648452

Beckman, H. B., & Frankel, R. M. (1994). The use of videotape in internal medicine training. *Journal of General Internal Medicine, 9*(9), 517–521. https://doi.org/10.1007/BF02599224

Beckman, H., Frankel, R., Kihm, J., Kulesza, G., & Geheb, M. (1990). Measurement and improvement of humanistic skills in first-year trainees. *Journal of General Internal Medicine, 5*(1), 42–45. https://doi.org/10.1007/BF02602308

Bell, C. M., & Redelmeier, D. A. (2001). Mortality among patients admitted to hospitals on weekends as compared with weekdays. *New England Journal of Medicine, 345*(9), 663–668. https://doi.org/10.1056/NEJMsa003376

Beňuš, Š., Gravano, A., & Hirschberg, J. (2011). Pragmatic aspects of temporal accommodation in turn-taking. *Journal of Pragmatics, 43*(12), 3001–3027. https://doi.org/10.1016/j.pragma.2011.05.011

Bidwell, J. T., Lyons, K. S., Mudd, J. O., Gelow, J. M., Chien, C. V., Hiatt, S. O., Grady, K. L., & Lee, C. S. (2017). Quality of life, depression, and anxiety in ventricular assist device therapy: Longitudinal outcomes for patients and family caregivers. *The Journal of Cardiovascular Nursing, 32*(5), 455–463. https://doi.org/10.1097/JCN.0000000000000378

Blanch, J. M. (2014). Quality of working life in commoditized hospitals and universities. *Iranian Journal of Public Health, 35*(1), 40–47.

Bochatay, N., & Bajwa, N. M. (2020). Learning to manage uncertainty: Supervision, trust and autonomy in residency training. *Sociology of Health & Illness, 42*(S1), 145–159. https://doi.org/10.1111/1467-9566.13070

Bohachick, P., Reeder, S., Taylor, M. V., & Anton, B. B. (2001). Psychosocial impact of heart transplantation on spouses. *Clinical Nursing Research, 10*(1), 6–25. https://doi.org/10.1177/c10n1r2

Bok, D. (2009). Universities in the marketplace. In *Universities in the marketplace.* Princeton University Press. https://www.degruyter.com/document/doi/10.1515/9781400825493/html

Bolden, G. B. (2009). Implementing incipient actions: The discourse marker 'so' in English conversation. *Journal of Pragmatics*, *41*(5), 974–998. https://doi.org/10. 1016/j.pragma.2008.10.004

Bourdieu, P. (1975). The specificity of the scientific field and the social conditions of the progress of reason. *Social Science Information*, *14*(6), 19–47. https://doi.org/ 10.1177/053901847501400602

Bourdieu, P. (1986). The forms of capital. In J. G. Richardson (Ed.), *Handbook of theory and research for the sociology of education* (pp. 241–258). Greenwood Press.

Bourdieu, P., & Wacquant, L. J. D. (1992). *An invitation to reflexive sociology*. University of Chicago Press.

Boyd, & Heritage, J. (2006). Taking the patient's medical history: Questioning during comprehensive history taking. In J. Heritage & D. W. Maynard (Eds.), *Communication in medical care: Interaction between primary care physicians and patients* (pp. 151–184). Cambridge University Press.

Bradac, J. J. (2001). Theory comparison: Uncertainty reduction, problematic integration, uncertainty management, and other curious constructs. *Journal of Communication*, *51*(3), 456–476. https://doi.org/10.1111/j.1460-2466.2001.tb02891.x

Braddock, C. H., Edwards, K. A., Hasenberg, N. M., Laidley, T. L., & Levinson, W. (1999). Informed decision making in outpatient practice: Time to get back to basics. *JAMA*, *282*(24), 2313–2320. https://doi.org/10.1001/jama.282.24.2313

Braddock, C. H., Fihn, S. D., Levinson, W., Jonsen, A. R., & Pearlman, R. A. (1997). How doctors and patients discuss routine clinical decisions. *Journal of General Internal Medicine*, *12*(6), 339–345. https://doi.org/10.1046/j.1525-1497.1997.00057.x

Braude, H. D. (2009). Clinical intuition versus statistics: Different modes of tacit knowledge in clinical epidemiology and evidence-based medicine. *Theoretical Medicine and Bioethics*, *30*(3), 181–198. https://doi.org/10.1007/s11017-009-9106-4

Brouwers, C., Denollet, J., de Jonge, N., Caliskan, K., Kealy, J., & Pedersen, S. S. (2011). Patient-reported outcomes in left ventricular assist device therapy. *Circulation: Heart Failure*, *4*(6), 714–723. https://doi.org/10.1161/CIRCHEARTFAILURE.111. 962472

Brun, W., Edland, A. C., Gärling, T., Harte, J. M., Hill, T., Huber, O., & Karlsson, N. (1997). *Decision making: Cognitive models and explanations*. Psychology Press.

Bullock, E. C. (2016). Mandatory disclosure and medical paternalism. *Ethical Theory and Moral Practice*, *19*(2), 409–424. https://doi.org/10.1007/s10677-015-9632-2

Bunzel, B., Laederach-Hofmann, G., Wieselthaler, W., Roethy, W., & Drees, G. (2005). Posttraumatic stress disorder after implantation of a mechanical assist device followed by heart transplantation: Evaluation of patients and partners. *Transplantation Proceedings*, *37*, 1365–1368.

Bunzel, B., Laederach-Hofmann, K., Wieselthaler, G., Roethy, W., & Wolner, E. (2007). Mechanical circulatory support as a bridge to heart transplantation: What remains? Long-term emotional sequelae in patients and spouses. *The Journal of Heart and Lung Transplantation*, *26*(4), 384–389. https://doi.org/10.1016/j.healun.2007.01.025

Burker, E. J., Evon, D., Loiselle, M. M., Finkel, J., & Mill, M. (2005). Planning helps, behavioral disengagement does not: Coping and depression in the spouses of heart transplant candidates. *Clinical Transplantation*, *19*(5), 653–658. https://doi.org/10. 1111/j.1399-0012.2005.00390.x

Butler, J. (1997). *The psychic life of power: Theories in subjection.* Stanford University Press.

Caldwell, P. H., Arthur, H. M., & Demers, C. (2007). Preferences of patients with heart failure for prognosis communication. *The Canadian Journal of Cardiology, 23*(10), 791–796.

Campbell, T., Schwarz, C., & Windschitl, M. (2016). What we call misconceptions may be necessary stepping-stones toward making sense of the world. *Science and Children, 53*(7), 28–33.

Canning, R. D., Dew, M. A., & Davidson, S. (1996). Psychological distress among caregivers to heart transplant recipients. *Social Science & Medicine, 42*(4), 599–608. https://doi.org/10.1016/0277-9536(95)00160-3

Chand, R., Lum, C. J., Chang, A., Salimbangon, A., Deng, M., Cadeiras, M., Khuu, T., Pandya, K., Vucicevic, D., Ardehali, A., & DePasquale, E. (2019). Is there a mortality "weekend effect" in cardiac transplantation? *The Journal of Heart and Lung Transplantation, 38*(4 Suppl), S396. https://doi.org/10.1016/j.healun.2019.01. 1008

Chodosh, S. (2018, December 11). The holiday season can be deadly for hospital patients. *Popular Science.* https://www.popsci.com/hospital-holiday-discharge-death/

Cicourel, A. V. (1987). The interpenetration of communicative contexts: Examples from medical encounters. In A. Duranti & C. Goodwin (Eds.), *Rethinking context: Language as an interactive phenomenon* (pp. 291–310).

Cicourel, A. V. (2011). Evidence and inference in macro-level and micro-level healthcare studies. In C. N. Candlin & S. Sarangi (Eds.), *Handbook of Communication in Organisations and Professions* (pp. 61–82). De Gruyter Mouton. https://doi.org/10. 1515/9783110214222.61

CNN. (2018, December 10). Holiday hospitalization carries higher risks, study says. In *CNN health.* CNN. https://www.cnn.com/2018/12/10/health/christmas-hospitalization-risks-study/index.html

Coates, J. (2013). One-at-a-time: The organisation of men's talk [1997]. In J. Coates (Ed.), *Women, men and everyday talk* (pp. 127–145). Palgrave Macmillan. https://doi.org/ 10.1057/9781137314949_7

Coates, J., & Sutton-Spence, R. (2001). Turn-taking patterns in deaf conversation. *Journal of Sociolinguistics, 5*(4), 507–529. https://doi.org/10.1111/1467-9481.00162

Cohen, A. M., Stavri, P. Z., & Hersh, W. R. (2004). A categorization and analysis of the criticisms of evidence-based medicine. *International Journal of Medical Informatics, 73*(1), 35–43. https://doi.org/10.1016/j.ijmedinf.2003.11.002

Conway, A., Schadewaldt, V., Clark, R., Ski, C., Thompson, D. R., & Doering, L. (2013). The psychological experiences of adult heart transplant recipients: A systematic review and meta-summary of qualitative findings. *Heart & Lung, 42*(6), 449–455. https://doi.org/10.1016/j.hrtlng.2013.08.003

Cooke, S., & Lemay, J.-F. (2017). Transforming medical assessment: Integrating uncertainty into the evaluation of clinical reasoning in medical education. *Academic Medicine, 92*(6), 746–751. https://doi.org/10.1097/ACM.0000000000001559

Cooper, L. T., Berry, G. J., & Shabetai, R. (1997). Idiopathic giant-cell myocarditis — Natural history and treatment. *New England Journal of Medicine, 336*(26), 1860–1866. https://doi.org/10.1056/NEJM199706263362603

Coopmans, C., Vertesi, J., Lynch, M. E., & Woolgar, S. (2014). *Representation in scientific practice revisited.* MIT Press.

Crossland, D. S., Van De Bruaene, A., Silversides, C. K., Hickey, E. J., & Roche, S. L. (2019). Heart failure in adult congenital heart disease: From advanced therapies to end-of-life care. *Canadian Journal of Cardiology, 35*(12), 1723–1739. https://doi. org/10.1016/j.cjca.2019.07.626

DeGroot, L. G., Bidwell, J. T., Peeler, A. C., Larsen, L. T., Davidson, P. M., & Abshire, M. A. (2021). "Talking around it": A qualitative study exploring dyadic congruence in managing the uncertainty of living with a ventricular assist device. *The Journal of Cardiovascular Nursing, 36*(3), 229–237. https://doi.org/10.1097/ JCN.0000000000000784

Deleuze, G., Guattari, F., & Massumi, B. (1980). *A thousand plateaus: Capitalism and schizophrenia.* https://doi.org/10.2307/203963

Delgado, J. F., Almenar, L., González-Vilchez, F., Arizón, J. M., Gómez, M., Fuente, L., Brossa, V., Fernández, J., Díaz, B., Pascual, D., Lage, E., Sanz, M., Manito, N., & Crespo-Leiro, M. G. (2015). Health-related quality of life, social support, and caregiver burden between six and 120 months after heart transplantation: A Spanish multicenter cross-sectional study. *Clinical Transplantation, 29*(9), 771–780. https://doi.org/10.1111/ctr.12578

Deng, M. C. & Naka, Y. Mechanical circulatory support therapy in advanced heart failure. World Scientific; 2007.

Deng, M. C. (2018). A peripheral blood transcriptome biomarker test to diagnose functional recovery potential in advanced heart failure. *Biomarkers in Medicine, 12*(6), 619–635. https://doi.org/10.2217/bmm-2018-0097

Deng, M. C. (2021). The evolution of patient-specific precision biomarkers to guide personalized heart-transplant care. *Expert Review of Precision Medicine and Drug Development, 6*(1), 51–63. https://doi.org/10.1080/23808993.2021.1840273

Deng, M. C., Eisen, H. J., Mehra, M. R., Billingham, M., Marboe, C. C., Berry, G., Kobashigawa, J., Johnson, F. L., Starling, R. C., Murali, S., Pauly, D. F., Baron, H., Wohlgemuth, J. G., Woodward, R. N., Klingler, T. M., Walther, D., Lal, P. G., Rosenberg, S., & Hunt, S. (2006). Noninvasive discrimination of rejection in cardiac allograft recipients using gene expression profiling. *American Journal of Transplantation, 6*(1), 150–160. https://doi.org/10.1111/j.1600-6143.2005.01175.x

Dew, M. A., Goycoolea, J. M., Stukas, A. A., Switzer, G. E., Simmons, R. G., Roth, L. H., & DiMartini, A. (1998). Temporal profiles of physical health in family members of heart transplant recipients: Predictors of health change during caregiving. *Health Psychology: Official Journal of the Division of Health Psychology, American Psychological Association, 17*(2), 138–151. https://doi.org/10.1037//0278-6133.17. 2.138

Dew, M. A., Kormos, R. L., Winowich, S., Harris, R. C., Stanford, E. A., Carozza, L., & Griffith, B. P. (2001). Quality of life outcomes after heart transplantation in individuals bridged to transplant with ventricular assist devices. *The Journal of Heart and Lung Transplantation, 20*(11), 1199–1212. https://doi.org/10.1016/ S1053-2498(01)00333-3

Dew, M. A., Myaskovsky, L., Dimartini, A. F., Switzer, G. E., Schulberg, H. C., & Kormos, R. L. (2004). Onset, timing and risk for depression and anxiety in family caregivers to heart transplant recipients. *Psychological Medicine, 34*(6), 1065–1082. https://doi.org/10.1017/S0033291703001387

Dreyfus, H. L., & Dreyfus, S. E. (1988). *Mind over machine: The power of human intuition and expertise in the era of the computer.* The Free Press.

Dube, G., Pastan, S., Patzer, R., & Mohan, S. (2014). Does transplant on the weekend affect outcomes following kidney transplant? A UNOS analysis: Abstract# C1864. *Transplantation, 98*, 599.

Duranti, A. (2005). Agency in language. In A. Duranti (Ed.), *A companion to linguistic anthropology* (1st ed., pp. 449–473). Wiley. https://doi.org/10.1002/9780470996522.ch20

ECC Committee, Subcommittees and Task Forces of the American Heart Association. (2005). 2005 American Heart Association Guidelines for Cardiopulmonary Resuscitation and Emergency Cardiovascular Care. *Circulation, 112*(Suppl. 24), IV1–203. https://doi.org/10.1161/CIRCULATIONAHA.105.166550

Eckman, M. H., Wise, R. E., Naylor, K., Arduser, L., Lip, G. Y. H., Kissela, B., Flaherty, M., Kleindorfer, D., Khan, F., Schauer, D. P., Kues, J., & Costea, A. (2015). Developing an Atrial Fibrillation Guideline Support Tool (AFGuST) for shared decision making. *Current Medical Research and Opinion, 31*(4), 603–614. https://doi.org/10.1185/03007995.2015.1019608

Edelsky, C. (1981). Who's got the floor? *Language in Society, 10*(3), 383–421. https://doi.org/10.1017/S004740450000885X

Elamm, C. A., Al-Kindi, S. G., Bianco, C. M., Dhakal, B. P., & Oliveira, G. H. (2017). Heart transplantation in giant cell myocarditis: Analysis of the United Network for Organ Sharing Registry. *Journal of Cardiac Failure, 23*(7), 566–569. https://doi.org/10.1016/j.cardfail.2017.04.015

Engelhardt, E. G., Pieterse, A. H., van der Hout, A., de Haes, H. J. C. J. M., Kroep, J. R., Quarles van Ufford-Mannesse, P., Portielje, J. E. A., Smets, E. M. A., & Stiggelbout, A. M. (2016). Use of implicit persuasion in decision making about adjuvant cancer treatment: A potential barrier to shared decision making. *European Journal of Cancer, 66*, 55–66. https://doi.org/10.1016/j.ejca.2016.07.011

Evangelista, L. S., Doering, L. V., Dracup, K., Vassilakis, M. E., & Kobashigawa, J. (2003). Hope, mood states and quality of life in female heart transplant recipients. *The Journal of Heart and Lung Transplantation, 22*(6), 681–686. https://doi.org/10.1016/S1053-2498(02)00652-6

Farnan, J. M., Johnson, J. K., Meltzer, D. O., Humphrey, H. J., & Arora, V. M. (2008). Resident uncertainty in clinical decision making and impact on patient care: A qualitative study. *BMJ Quality & Safety, 17*(2), 122–126. https://doi.org/10.1136/qshc.2007.023184

Feinstein, A. R., & Horwitz, R. I. (1997). Problems in the "evidence" of "evidence-based medicine." *The American Journal of Medicine, 103*(6), 529–535. https://doi.org/10.1016/s0002-9343(97)00244-1

Foucault, M. (1977). *Discipline and Punish: The Birth of the Prison.* Random House.

Foucault, M. (1990). *The history of sexuality: An introduction.* Vintage Books.

Fox, R. C. (1957). Training for uncertainty. In R. K. Merton, G. G. Reader, & P. Kendall (Eds.), *The student-physician* (pp. 207–240). Harvard University Press. https://www.hup.harvard.edu/catalog.php?isbn$=$9780674366831

Fox, R. C. (1980). The evolution of medical uncertainty. *The Milbank Memorial Fund Quarterly Health and Society, 58*(1), 1–49.

Fox, R. C. (2003). Medical uncertainty revisited. In G. L. Albrecht, R. Fitzpatrick, & S. C. Scrimshaw (Eds.), *The handbook of social studies in health and medicine* (pp. 409–425). Sage.

Fox, R. C., & Swazey, J. P. (1974a). *The courage to fail: A social view of organ transplants and dialysis.* University of Chicago Press.

Fox, R. C., & Swazey, J. P. (1974b). *The courage to fail: A social view of organ transplants and dialysis.* Monograph Collection (Matt-Pseudo).

Frankel, R. M. (1983). The laying on of hands: Aspects of the organization of gaze, touch, and talk in a medical encounter. In *The social organization of doctor-patient communication* (pp. 19–54).

Frankel, R. M. (1984). From sentence to sequence: Understanding the medical encounter through microinteractional analysis. *Discourse Processes, 7*(2), 135–170. https://doi.org/10.1080/01638538409544587

Frankel, R. M., & Beckman, H. B. (1982). Impact: An interaction-based method for preserving and analyzing clinical transactions. In *Explorations in Provider and Patient Interactions* (pp. 71–85).

Frankel, R. M., & Beckman, H. B. (2017). Physicians interrupting patients. *JAMA, 318*(1), 93–93. https://doi.org/10.1001/jama.2017.6489

Garfinkel, H., & Harvey Sacks. (1970). On formal structures of practical actions. In J. C. McKinney & Edward A. Tiryakian (Eds.), *Theoretical sociology: Perspectives and developments* (pp. 337–366). Appleton-Century-Crofts.

Geller, G., Faden, R. R., & Levine, D. M. (1990). Tolerance for ambiguity among medical students: Implications for their selection, training and practice. *Social Science & Medicine, 31*(5), 619–624. https://doi.org/10.1016/0277-9536(90)90098-D

Geller, G., Grbic, D., Andolsek, K. M., Caulfield, M., & Roskovensky, L. (2021). Tolerance for ambiguity among medical students: Patterns of change during medical school and their implications for professional development. *Academic Medicine, 96*(7), 1036–1042. https://doi.org/10.1097/ACM.0000000000003820

Geller, G., Tambor, E. S., Chase, G. A., & Holtzman, N. A. (1993). Measuring physicians' tolerance for ambiguity and its relationship to their reported practices regarding genetic testing. *Medical Care, 31*(11), 989–1001.

Gherardi, S. (2009). Introduction: The critical power of the 'Practice Lens'. *Management Learning, 40*(2), 115–128. https://doi.org/10.1177/1350507608101225

Gill, V. T., & Robert, F. (2013). Conversation analysis in medicine. In J. Sidnell & T. Stivers (Eds.), *The handbook of conversation analysis* (pp. 575–592). Wiley-Blackwell.

Gishen, F. (2020). *Evaluating a curriculum map for undergraduate medical education: A critical analysis through different stakeholder lenses.* [Doctoral thesis, University College London]. https://discovery.ucl.ac.uk/id/eprint/10114422/

Goffman, E. (1959). *The presentation of self in everyday life.* Doubleday.

Goffman, E. (1974). *Frame analysis: An essay on the organization of experience* (pp. ix, 586). Harvard University Press.

Goffman, E. (1981). *Forms of talk.* University of Pennsylvania Press.

Goldenberg, M. J. (2006). On evidence and evidence-based medicine: Lessons from the philosophy of science. *Social Science & Medicine, 62*(11), 2621–2632. https://doi.org/10.1016/j.socscimed.2005.11.031

Gonzalo, J. D., Kuperman, E., Lehman, E., & Haidet, P. (2014). Bedside interprofessional rounds: Perceptions of benefits and barriers by internal medicine nursing staff, attending physicians, and housestaff physicians. *Journal of Hospital Medicine, 9*(10), 646–651. https://doi.org/10.1002/jhm.2245

Goodlin, S. J., Hauptman, P. J., Arnold, R., Grady, K., Hershberger, R. E., Kutner, J., Masoudi, F., Spertus, J., Dracup, K., Cleary, J. F., Medak, R., Crispell, K., piña, I., Stuart, B., Whitney, C., Rector, T., Teno, J., & Renlund, D. G. (2004). Consensus statement: Palliative and supportive care in advanced heart failure. *Journal of Cardiac Failure, 10*(3), 200–209. https://doi.org/10.1016/j.cardfail.2003.09.006

Goodwin, C. (1986). Between and within: Alternative sequential treatments of continuers and assessments. *Human Studies, 9*(2–3), 205–217. https://doi.org/10.1007/BF00148127

Goodwin, C. (1994). Professional vision. *American Anthropologist, 96*(3), 606–633. https://doi.org/10.1525/aa.1994.96.3.02a00100

Goodwin, C. (2000a). Action and embodiment within situated human interaction. *Journal of Pragmatics, 32*, 1489–1522.

Goodwin, C. (2000b). Action and embodiment within situated human interaction. *Journal of Pragmatics, 32*(10), 1489–1522. https://doi.org/10.1016/S0378-2166(99)00096-X

Goodwin, C. (2017). *Co-operative action: Learning in doing. Social, cognitive & computational perspectives.* Cambridge University Press.

Goodwin, C. (2018). *Co-operative action.* Cambridge University Press.

Goodwin, C., & Duranti, A. (1992). Rethinking context: An introduction. In A. Duranti & C. Goodwin (Eds.), *Rethinking context: Language as an interactive phenomenon.* Cambridge University Press.

Goodwin, C., & Goodwin, M. H. (1997). Contested vision: The discursive constitution of Rodney King. In B. L. Gunnarsson, P. Linell, & B. Nordberg (Eds.), *The construction of professional discourse* (pp. 292–316). Routledge.

Goodwin, M. H. (1980). Processes of mutual monitoring implicated in the production of description sequences. *Sociological Inquiry, 50*(3–4), 303–317. https://doi.org/10.1111/j.1475-682X.1980.tb00024.x

Goodwin, M. H. (1996). Shifting frame. In D. I. Slobin, J. Gerhardt, A. Kyratzis, & J. Guo (Eds.), *Social interaction, social context, and language: Essays in honor of Susan Ervin-tripp* (pp. 71–82). Psychology Press.

Goodwin, M. H., & Cekaite, A. (2018). *Embodied family choreography: Practices of control, care, and mundane creativity.* Routledge.

Goodwin, M. H., & Goodwin, C. (2000). Emotion within situated activity. In N. Budwig, I. Č. Užgiris, & J. V. Wertsch (Eds.), *Communication: An arena of development* (pp. 33–53).

Goodwin, M., & Cekaite, A. (2013). Calibration in directive/response sequences in family interaction. *Journal of Pragmatics, 46*(1 SRC-GoogleScholar), 122–138.

Goodwin, M., & Language Discourse. (2006). Participation, affect, and trajectory in family directive/response sequences. *Text Talk An Interdisciplinary Journal of Studies No 515543, 26*(SRC-Google Scholar), 4–5.

Grant, E. V., Summapund, J., Matlock, D. D., Vaughan Dickson, V., Iqbal, S., Patel, S., Katz, S. D., Chaudhry, S. I., & Dodson, J. A. (2020). Patient and cardiologist perspectives on shared decision making in the treatment of older adults hospitalized for acute myocardial infarction. *Medical Decision Making, 40*(3), 279–288. https://doi.org/10.1177/0272989X20912293

Greenhalgh, T., Snow, R., Ryan, S., Rees, S., & Salisbury, H. (2015). Six 'biases' against patients and carers in evidence-based medicine. *BMC Medicine, 13*(1), 200. https://doi.org/10.1186/s12916-015-0437-x

Haddow, G. (2005). The phenomenology of death, embodiment and organ transplantation. *Sociology of Health & Illness, 27*(1), 92–113. https://doi.org/10.1111/j.1467-9566.2005.00433.x

Hall, R., & Stevens, R. (2015). Interaction analysis approaches to knowledge in use. In A. A. diSessa, M. Levin, & N. J. S. Brown (Eds.), *Knowledge and interaction: A synthetic agenda for the learning sciences* (pp. 72–108). Routledge.

Han, P. K. J., Babrow, A., Hillen, M. A., Gulbrandsen, P., Smets, E. M., & Ofstad, E. H. (2019). Uncertainty in health care: Towards a more systematic program of research. *Patient Education and Counseling, 102*(10), 1756–1766. https://doi.org/10.1016/j.pec.2019.06.012

Han, P. K. J., Klein, W. M. P., & Arora, N. K. (2011). Varieties of uncertainty in health care: A conceptual taxonomy. *Medical Decision Making, 31*(6), 828–838. https://doi.org/10.1177/0272989X10393976

Han, P. K. J., Schupack, D., Daggett, S., Holt, C. T., & Strout, T. D. (2015a). Temporal changes in tolerance of uncertainty among medical students: Insights from an exploratory study. *Medical Education Online, 20*(1), 28285. https://doi.org/10.3402/meo.v20.28285

Han, P. K. J., Schupack, D., Daggett, S., Holt, C. T., & Strout, T. D. (2015b). Temporal changes in tolerance of uncertainty among medical students: Insights from an exploratory study. *Medical Education Online, 20*(1), 28285. https://doi.org/10.3402/meo.v20.28285

Han, P. K. J., Strout, T. D., Gutheil, C., Germann, C., King, B., Ofstad, E., Gulbrandsen, P., & Trowbridge, R. (2021). How physicians manage medical uncertainty: A qualitative study and conceptual taxonomy. *Medical Decision Making, 41*(3), 275–291. https://doi.org/10.1177/0272989X21992340

Hargraves, I., LeBlanc, A., Shah, N. D., & Montori, V. M. (2016). Shared decision making: The need for patient-clinician conversation, not just information. *Health Affairs, 35*(4), 627–629. https://doi.org/10.1377/hlthaff.2015.1354

Healy, K. (2006). *Last best gifts: Altruism and the market for human blood and organs* (pp. xiii, 193). University of Chicago Press. https://doi.org/10.7208/chicago/9780226322384.001.0001

Heath, C. (1986). *Body movement and speech in medical interaction.* Cambridge University Press.

Heath, C. (1988). Embarrassment and interactional organization. In P. Drew & A. Wootton (Eds.), *Erving Goffman: Exploring the interaction order* (Vols. 136–150). Polity Press, Northeastern University Press Boston.

Heath, C., & Luff, P. (2007). Gesture and institutional interaction: Figuring bids in auctions of fine art and antiques. *Gesture, 7*(2), 215–240. https://doi.org/10.1075/gest.7.2.05hea

Hedley, J. A., Chang, N., Kelly, P. J., Rosales, B. M., Wyburn, K., O'Leary, M., Cavazzoni, E., & Webster, A. C. (2019). Weekend effect: Analysing temporal trends in solid organ donation. *ANZ Journal of Surgery*, *89*(9), 1068–1074. https://doi.org/10.1111/ans.15015

Heidegger, M. (1976, May 31). Only a god can save us. *Der Spiegel*, *23*, 193–219.

Helft, P. R. (2005). Necessary collusion: Prognostic communication with advanced cancer patients. *Journal of Clinical Oncology*, *23*(13), 3146–3150. https://doi.org/10.1200/JCO.2005.07.003

Henry, S., Zaner, R., & Dittus, R. (2007). Viewpoint: Moving beyond evidence-based medicine. *Academic Medicine, 82*(3), 292–297. https://doi.org/10.1097/ACM.0b013e3180307f6d

Heritage, J. (2010). Questioning in medicine. In A. Freed & S. Ehrlich (Eds.), *Why do you ask?: The function of questions in institutional discourse* (pp. 42–68). Oxford University Press.

Heritage, J., & Atkinson, J. M. (1984). Introduction. In J. M. Atkinson & J. Heritage (Eds.), *Structures of social action: Studies in conversation analysis*. Cambridge University Press.

Heritage, J., & Maynard, D. W. (2006). *Communication in medical care: Interaction between primary care physicians and patients*. Cambridge University Press.

Hess, E. P., Grudzen, C. R., Thomson, R., Raja, A. S., & Carpenter, C. R. (2015). Shared decision-making in the emergency department: Respecting patient autonomy when seconds count. *Academic Emergency Medicine, 22*(7), 856–864. https://doi.org/10.1111/acem.12703

Hillen, M. A., Gutheil, C. M., Strout, T. D., Smets, E. M. A., & Han, P. K. J. (2017). Tolerance of uncertainty: Conceptual analysis, integrative model, and implications for healthcare. *Social Science & Medicine (1982), 180*, 62–75. https://doi.org/10.1016/j.socscimed.2017.03.024

Hindmarsh, J., & Pilnick, A. (2002). The tacit order of teamwork: Collaboration and embodied conduct in anesthesia. *Sociological Quarterly, 43*(2), 139–164. https://doi.org/10.1111/j.1533-8525.2002.tb00044.x

Hjørland, B. (2011). Evidence-based practice: An analysis based on the philosophy of science. *Journal of the American Society for Information Science and Technology, 62*(7), 1301–1310. https://doi.org/10.1002/asi.21523

Holt, E. (1993). The structure of death announcements: Looking on the bright side of death. *Text-Interdisciplinary Journal for the Study of Discourse, 13*(2), 189–212. https://doi.org/10.1515/text.1.1993.13.2.189

Horwitz, R. I. (1996). The dark side of evidence-based medicine. *Cleveland Clinic Journal of Medicine, 63*(6), 320–323.

Hunter, D. J. (2016). Uncertainty in the era of precision medicine. *New England Journal of Medicine, 375*(8), 711–713. https://doi.org/10.1056/NEJMp1608282

Ilgen, J. S., Eva, K. W., de Bruin, A., Cook, D. A., & Regehr, G. (2019). Comfort with uncertainty: Reframing our conceptions of how clinicians navigate complex clinical situations. *Advances in Health Sciences Education, 24*(4), 797–809. https://doi.org/10.1007/s10459-018-9859-5

Ivarsson, B., Ekmehag, B., & Sjöberg, T. (2014). Relative's experiences before and after a heart or lung transplantation. *Heart & Lung, 43*(3), 198–203. https://doi.org/10.1016/j.hrtlng.2014.02.005

Jefferson, G. (2004). Glossary of transcript symbols with an introduction. *Pragmatics and Beyond New Series, 125*, 13–34.

Jordan, B., & Henderson, A. (1995). Interaction analysis: Foundations and practice. *Journal of the Learning Sciences, 4*(1), 39–103. https://doi.org/10.1207/s15327809jls0401_2

Joseph-Williams, N., Elwyn, G., & Edwards, A. (2014). Knowledge is not power for patients: A systematic review and thematic synthesis of patient-reported barriers and facilitators to shared decision making. *Patient Education and Counseling, 94*(3), 291–309. https://doi.org/10.1016/j.pec.2013.10.031

Karnieli-Miller, O., & Eisikovits, Z. (2009). Physician as partner or salesman? Shared decision-making in real-time encounters. *Social Science & Medicine, 69*(1), 1–8. https://doi.org/10.1016/j.socscimed.2009.04.030

Kasper, J., Geiger, F., Freiberger, S., & Schmidt, A. (2008). Decision-related uncertainties perceived by people with cancer — Modelling the subject of shared decision making. *Psycho-Oncology, 17*(1), 42–48. https://doi.org/10.1002/pon.1190

Kirklin, J. K., Naftel, D. C., Pagani, F. D., Kormos, R. L., Stevenson, L. W., Blume, E. D., Myers, S. L., Miller, M. A., Baldwin, J. T., & Young, J. B. (2015). Seventh INTERMACS annual report: 15,000 patients and counting. *The Journal of Heart and Lung Transplantation, 34*(12), 1495–1504. https://doi.org/10.1016/j.healun.2015.10.003

Kitko, L. A., Hupcey, J. E., Pinto, C., & Palese, M. (2015). Patient and Caregiver incongruence in advanced heart failure. *Clinical Nursing Research, 24*(4), 388–400. https://doi.org/10.1177/1054773814523777

Kitko, L., McIlvennan, C. K., Bidwell, J. T., Dionne-Odom, J. N., Dunlay, S. M., Lewis, L. M., Meadows, G., Sattler, E. L. P., Schulz, R., Strömberg, A., American Heart Association Council on Cardiovascular and Stroke Nursing, Council on Quality of Care and Outcomes Research, Council on Clinical Cardiology, & Council on Lifestyle and Cardiometabolic Health. (2020). Family caregiving for individuals with heart failure: A scientific statement from the American heart association. *Circulation, 141*(22), e864–e878. https://doi.org/10.1161/CIR.0000000000000768

Klindtworth, K., Oster, P., Hager, K., Krause, O., Bleidorn, J., & Schneider, N. (2015). Living with and dying from advanced heart failure: Understanding the needs of older patients at the end of life. *BMC Geriatrics, 15*, 125. https://doi.org/10.1186/s12877-015-0124-y

Knight, L. V., & Mattick, K. (2006). 'When I first came here, I thought medicine was black and white': Making sense of medical students' ways of knowing. *Social Science & Medicine, 63*(4), 1084–1096. https://doi.org/10.1016/j.socscimed.2006.01.017

Köllner, V., Schade, I., Maulhardt, T., Maercker, A., Joraschky, P., & Gulielmos, V. (2002). Posttraumatic stress disorder and quality of life after heart or lung transplantation. *Transplantation Proceedings, 34*(6), 2192–2193. https://doi.org/10.1016/S0041-1345(02)03198-6

Koschmann, T., & LeBaron, C. (2002). Learner articulation as interactional achievement: studying the conversation of gesture. *Cognition and Instruction, 20*(2), 249–282. https://doi.org/10.1207/S1532690XCI2002_4

Koschmann, T., LeBaron, C., Goodwin, C., & Feltovich, P. (2011). "Can you see the cystic artery yet?" A simple matter of trust. *Journal of Pragmatics, 43*(2), 521–541. https://doi.org/10.1016/j.pragma.2009.09.009

Kostick, K. M., Bruce, C. R., Minard, C. G., Volk, R. J., Civitello, A., Krim, S. R., Horstmanshof, D., Thohan, V., Loebe, M., Hanna, M., Bruckner, B. A., Blumenthal-Barby, J. S., & Estep, J. D. (2018). A multisite randomized controlled trial of a patient-centered ventricular assist device decision aid (VADDA Trial). *Journal of Cardiac Failure, 24*(10), 661–671. https://doi.org/10.1016/j.cardfail.2018.08.008

Kostick, K., Trejo, M., & Blumenthal-Barby, J. S. (2019). Suffering and healing in the context of LVAD treatment. *Journal of Clinical Medicine, 8*(5), 660. https://doi.org/10.3390/jcm8050660

Kuhn, G., Goldberg, R., & Compton, S. (2009). Tolerance for uncertainty, burnout, and satisfaction with the career of emergency medicine. *Annals of Emergency Medicine, 54*(1), 106–113.e6. https://doi.org/10.1016/j.annemergmed.2008.12.019

Kunneman, M., Gionfriddo, M. R., Toloza, F. J. K., Gärtner, F. R., Spencer-Bonilla, G., Hargraves, I. G., Erwin, P. J., & Montori, V. M. (2019). Humanistic communication in the evaluation of shared decision making: A systematic review. *Patient Education and Counseling, 102*(3), 452–466. https://doi.org/10.1016/j.pec.2018.11.003

Latour, B. (1996). *On actor-network theory: A few clarifications* (pp. 369–381).

Lefaiver, C. A. (2006). *Quality of life: The dyad of caregivers and lung transplant candidates.* PhD dissertation, Loyola University, Chicago. https://search.proquest.com/docview/305300093/abstract/34C9D9E7C79D44ACPQ/1

Légaré, F., Ratté, S., Gravel, K., & Graham, I. D. (2008). Barriers and facilitators to implementing shared decision-making in clinical practice: Update of a systematic review of health professionals' perceptions. *Patient Education and Counseling, 73*(3), 526–535. https://doi.org/10.1016/j.pec.2008.07.018

Lévinas, E. (1969). *Totality and infinity: An essay on exteriority.* Duquesne University Press.

Lévinas, E., & Nemo, P. (1985). *Ethics and Infinity.*

Li, M., & Chapman, G. B. (2020). Medical decision making. In *The Wiley Encyclopedia of Health Psychology* (pp. 347–353). Wiley. https://doi.org/10.1002/9781119057840.ch84

Linell, P., & Bredmar, M. (1996). Reconstructing topical sensitivity: Aspects of face-work in talks between midwives and expectant mothers. *Research on Language & Social Interaction, 29*(4), 347–379. https://doi.org/10.1207/s15327973rlsi2904_3

Llewellyn, N., & Hindmarsh, J. (Eds.). (2010). *Organisation, interaction and practice: Studies in ethnomethodology and conversation analysis.* Cambridge University Press.

Lock, M. M. (2002). *Twice dead: Organ transplants and the reinvention of death.* University of California Press.

LoMauro, A., & Aliverti, A. (2018). Blood shift during cough: Negligible or significant? *Frontiers in Physiology, 9*, 501. https://doi.org/10.3389/fphys.2018.00501

Lumish, H. S., Clerkin, K. J., Marboe, C., Han, J., Latif, F., Restaino, S. W., Farr, M. A., Lin, E. F., Takayama, H., Takeda, K., Naka, Y., Colombo, P. C., & Yuzefpolskaya, M. (2018). (1093)-Giant cell myocarditis patients undergoing heart transplantation have high rates of rejection, infection and cardiac allograft Vasculopathy: Case series. *The Journal of Heart and Lung Transplantation, 37*(Suppl. 4), S422–S423. https://doi.org/10.1016/j.healun.2018.01.1096

Luna, M. J. (2018). What does it mean to notice my students' ideas in science today?: An investigation of elementary teachers' practice of noticing their students' thinking in science. *Cognition and Instruction, 36*(4), 297–329. https://doi.org/10.1080/07370008.2018.1496919

Lutfey, K., & Maynard, D. W. (1998). Bad news in oncology: How physician and patient talk about death and dying without using those words. *Social Psychology Quarterly, 61*(4), 321. https://doi.org/10.2307/2787033

Luther, V. P., & Crandall, S. J. (2011). Commentary: Ambiguity and uncertainty: Neglected elements of medical education curricula? *Academic Medicine, 86*(7), 799–800. https://doi.org/10.1097/ACM.0b013e31821da915

Lynch, M., & Woolgar, S. (1990). *Representation in scientific practice*. https://ora.ox.ac.uk/objects/uuid:88d240b7-3b6a-42af-b3db-e4effeb5925c

Magasi, S., Buono, S., Yancy, C. W., Ramirez, R. D., & Grady, K. L. (2019). Preparedness and mutuality affect quality of life for patients with mechanical circulatory support and their caregivers. *Circulation: Cardiovascular Quality and Outcomes, 12*(1), e004414. https://doi.org/10.1161/CIRCOUTCOMES.117.004414

Makdisi, G., & Wang, I. (2015). Extra corporeal membrane oxygenation (ECMO) review of a lifesaving technology. *Journal of Thoracic Disease, 7*(7), E166–E176. https://doi.org/10.3978/j.issn.2072-1439.2015.07.17

Marcuccilli, L., Casida, J. J., Bakas, T., & Pagani, F. D. (2014). Family caregivers' inside perspectives: Caring for an adult with a left ventricular assist device as a destination therapy. *Progress in Transplantation (Aliso Viejo, Calif.), 24*(4), 332–340. https://doi.org/10.7182/pit2014684

Mattingly, C. (1998). *Healing dramas and clinical plots: The narrative structure of experience*. Cambridge University Press.

Mauss, M. (2000). *The gift: The form and reason for exchange in archaic societies*. W. W. Norton & Company.

Mauthner, O., De Luca, E., Poole, J., Gewarges, M., Abbey, S. E., Shildrick, M., & Ross, H. (2012). Preparation and support of patients through the transplant process: Understanding the recipients' perspectives [Research article]. *Nursing Research and Practice, 2021*, 547312. https://doi.org/10.1155/2012/547312

Mauthner, O. E., De Luca, E., Poole, J. M., Abbey, S. E., Shildrick, M., Gewarges, M., & Ross, H. J. (2015a). Heart transplants: Identity disruption, bodily integrity and interconnectedness. *Health, 19*(6), 578–594. https://doi.org/10.1177/1363459314560067

Mauthner, O. E., De Luca, E., Poole, J. M., Abbey, S. E., Shildrick, M., Gewarges, M., & Ross, H. J. (2015b). Heart transplants: Identity disruption, bodily integrity and interconnectedness. *Health, 19*(6), 578–594. https://doi.org/10.1177/1363459314560067

Maynard, D. (1992). *On clinicians co-implicating recipients' Perspective in the delivery of diagnostic news*.

Maynard, D. W. (1991). Interaction and asymmetry in clinical discourse. *American Journal of Sociology, 97*(2), 448–495. https://doi.org/10.1086/229785

Maynard, D. W. (2003). *Bad news, Good news: Conversational order in everyday talk and clinical settings*. University of Chicago Press.

McClimans, L., & Slowther, A. (2016). Moral expertise in the clinic: Lessons learned from medicine and science. *The Journal of Medicine and Philosophy: A Forum for Bioethics and Philosophy of Medicine, 41*(4), 401–415. https://doi.org/10.1093/jmp/jhw011

McIlvennan, C. K., Matlock, D. D., Thompson, J. S., Dunlay, S. M., Blue, L., LaRue, S. J., Lewis, E. F., Patel, C. B., Fairclough, D. L., Leister, E. C., Swetz, K. M., Baldridge, V., Walsh, M. N., & Allen, L. A. (2018). Caregivers of patients considering a destination therapy left ventricular assist device and a shared decision-making intervention. *JACC: Heart Failure, 6*(11), 904–913. https://doi.org/10.1016/j.jchf.2018.06.019

McLemore, C. (1991). The interpretation of L* H in English. *Texas Linguistic Forum-Discourse, 32.*

Mclemore, C. A. (1992). *The pragmatic interpretation of English intonation: Sorority speech* (p. 1).

McNutt, R. A. (2004). Shared medical decision making: Problems, process, progress. *JAMA, 292*(20), 2516–2518. https://doi.org/10.1001/jama.292.20.2516

Menghini, V. V., Savcenko, V., Olson, L. J., Tazelaar, H. D., William Dec, G., Kao, A., & Cooper, L. T. (1999). Combined immuno suppression for the treatment of idiopathic giant cell myocarditis. *Mayo Clinic Proceedings, 74*(12), 1221–1226. https://doi.org/10.4065/74.12.1221

Merleau-Ponty, M. (1962). *Phenomenology of perception* (C. Smith, Trans.). Routledge & Kegan Paul.

Meyer, J. W. (2010). World Society, Institutional Theories, and the Actor. *Annual Review of Sociology, 36*(1), 1–20. https://doi.org/10.1146/annurev.soc.012809.102506

Mihalj, M., Carrel, T., Urman, R. D., Stueber, F., & Luedi, M. M. (2020). Recommendations for preoperative assessment and shared decision-making in cardiac surgery. *Current Anesthesiology Reports, 10*(2), 185–195. https://doi.org/10.1007/s40140-020-00377-7

Miles, A. (2009). Evidence-based medicine: Requiescat in pace? A commentary on Djulbegovic, B., Guyatt, G. H. & Ashcroft, R. E. (2009) Cancer Control, 16, 158–168. *Journal of Evaluation in Clinical Practice, 15*(6), 924–929. https://doi.org/10.1111/j.1365-2753.2009.01349.x

Minsky, M. (1975). A framework for representing knowledge. In P. Winston, Ed., *The Psychology of Computer Vision.* New York: McGraw-Hill, pp. 211–277.

Mishel, M. H. (1988). Uncertainty in Illness. *Image: The Journal of Nursing Scholarship, 20*(4), 225–232. https://doi.org/10.1111/j.1547-5069.1988.tb00082.x

Mishler, E. G. (1984). *The discourse of medicine: Dialectics of medical interviews.* Greenwood Publishing Group.

Mishler, E. G. (1997). The interactional construction of narratives in medical and life-history interviews. In B. L. Gunnarsson, P. Linell, & B. Nordberg (Eds.), *The construction of professional discourse* (pp. 223–244). Routledge.

Miyazaki, E. T., Santos, R. dos, Miyazaki, M. C., Domingos, N. M., Felicio, H. C., Rocha, M. F., Arroyo, P. C., Duca, W. J., Silva, R. F., & Silva, R. C. M. A. (2010). Patients on the waiting list for liver transplantation: Caregiver burden and stress. *Liver Transplantation, 16*(10), 1164–1168. https://doi.org/10.1002/lt.22130

Moayedi, Y., Ross, H. J., & Khush, K. K. (2018). Disclosure of infectious risk to heart transplant candidates: Shared decision-making is here to stay. *The Journal of Heart and Lung Transplantation, 37*(5), 564–567. https://doi.org/10.1016/j.healun.2017.12.014

Mondada, L. (2011). The organization of concurrent courses of action in surgical demonstrations. In J. Streeck, C. Goodwin, & C. LeBaron (Eds.), *Embodied interaction: Language and body in the material world* (pp. 207–226).

Moore, K., Kleinman, D. L., Hess, D., & Frickel, S. (2011). Science and neoliberal globalization: A political sociological approach. *Theory and Society, 40*(5), 505–532. https://doi.org/10.1007/s11186-011-9147-3

Morris, C., & Blaney, D. (2013). Work-based learning. In *Understanding medical education* (pp. 97–109). Wiley. https://doi.org/10.1002/9781118472361.ch7

Morris, R. S., Ruck, J. M., Conca-Cheng, A. M., Smith, T. J., Carver, T. W., & Johnston, F. M. (2018). Shared decision-making in acute surgical illness: The surgeon's perspective. *Journal of the American College of Surgeons, 226*(5), 784–795. https://doi.org/10.1016/j.jamcollsurg.2018.01.008

Napp, L. C., Kühn, C., Hoeper, M. M., Vogel-Claussen, J., Haverich, A., Schäfer, A., & Bauersachs, J. (2016). Cannulation strategies for percutaneous extracorporeal membrane oxygenation in adults. *Clinical Research in Cardiology, 105*(4), 283–296. https://doi.org/10.1007/s00392-015-0941-1

Nevalainen, M. K., Mantyranta, T., & Pitkala, K. H. (2010). Facing uncertainty as a medical student — A qualitative study of their reflective learning diaries and writings on specific themes during the first clinical year. *Patient Education and Counseling, 78*(2), 218–223. https://doi.org/10.1016/j.pec.2009.07.011

Nicolini, D. (2006). The work to make telemedicine work: A social and articulative view. *Social Science & Medicine, 62*(11), 2754–2767. https://doi.org/10.1016/j.socscimed.2005.11.001

Nicolini, D. (2010). Medical innovation as a process of translation: A case from the field of telemedicine. *British Journal of Management, 21*(4), 1011–1026. https://doi.org/10.1111/j.1467-8551.2008.00627.x

Nicolini, D. (2012). *Practice theory, work, and organization: An introduction.* OUP Oxford.

Noonan, M. C., Wingham, J., & Taylor, R. S. (2018). 'Who cares?' The experiences of caregivers of adults living with heart failure, chronic obstructive pulmonary disease and coronary artery disease: A mixed methods systematic review. *BMJ Open, 8*(7), e020927. https://doi.org/10.1136/bmjopen-2017-020927

Numerato, D., Salvatore, D., & Fattore, G. (2012). The impact of management on medical professionalism: A review. *Sociology of Health & Illness, 34*(4), 626–644. https://doi.org/10.1111/j.1467-9566.2011.01393.x

Nye, J. S. (2004). *Soft power: The means to success in world politics.* Public Affairs.

Nye, J. S. (2008). Public diplomacy and soft power. *The ANNALS of the American Academy of Political and Social Science, 616*(1), 94–109. https://doi.org/10.1177/0002716207311699

Ochs, E. (1979). Transcription as theory. *Developmental Pragmatics, 10*(1), 43–72.

Ochs, E., & Schieffelin, B. (2009). Language has a heart. *Text-Interdisciplinary Journal for the Study of Discourse, 9*(1), 7–26. https://doi.org/10.1515/text.1.1989.9.1.7

Ogden, R. (2006). Phonetics and social action in agreements and disagreements. *Journal of Pragmatics, 38*(10), 1752–1775. https://doi.org/10.1016/j.pragma.2005.04.011

Paradis, E., Leslie, M., & Gropper, M. A. (2016). Interprofessional rhetoric and operational realities: An ethnographic study of rounds in four intensive care units. *Advances in Health Sciences Education, 21*(4), 735–748. https://doi.org/10.1007/s10459-015-9662-5

Parascandola, M., Hawkins, J. S., & Danis, M. (2002). Patient autonomy and the challenge of clinical uncertainty. *Kennedy Institute of Ethics Journal, 12*(3), 245–264. https://doi.org/10.1353/ken.2002.0018

Parry, R. (2018). *Distribution of agency across body and self.* Loughborough University. https://repository.lboro.ac.uk/articles/Distribution_of_agency_across_body_and_self/9478868

Parsons, T. (1951). Social Structure and Dynamic Process: The Case of Modern Medical Practice. The Social System, chapter 10, 428–479, Glencoe, 111.: Free Press

Parsons, T. (2013). Structure and Dynamic Process: The Case of Modern Medical Practice in *The Social System*. Chapter 10, Routledge, pg 228–232

Pellegrino, E. D. (1999). The commodification of medical and health care: The moral consequences of a paradigm shift from a professional to a market ethic. *The Journal of Medicine and Philosophy: A Forum for Bioethics and Philosophy of Medicine, 24*(3), 243–266. https://doi.org/10.1076/jmep.24.3.243.2523

Peters, M., & ten Cate, O. (2014). Bedside teaching in medical education: A literature review. *Perspectives on Medical Education, 3*(2), 76–88. https://doi.org/10.1007/s40037-013-0083-y

Pieterse, A. H., Stiggelbout, A. M., & Montori, V. M. (2019). Shared decision making and the importance of time. *JAMA, 322*(1), 25–26. https://doi.org/10.1001/jama.2019.3785

Politi, M. C., Han, P. K. J., & Col, N. F. (2007). Communicating the uncertainty of harms and benefits of medical interventions. *Medical Decision Making, 27*(5), 681–695. https://doi.org/10.1177/0272989X07307270

Pomerantz, A. (1984). In J. M. Atkinson & J. Heritage (Eds.), *Agreeing and disagreeing with assessments: Some features of preferred/dispreferred turn shaped* (pp. 57–101).

Punjabi, P. P., & Taylor, K. M. (2013). The science and practice of cardiopulmonary bypass: From cross circulation to ECMO and SIRS. *Global Cardiology Science & Practice, 2013*(3), 249–260. https://doi.org/10.5339/gcsp.2013.32

Raia, F. (2018). Identity, tools and existential spaces. *Learning, Culture and Social Interaction, 19*, 74–95. https://doi.org/10.1016/j.lcsi.2018.04.014

Raia, F. (2020). The temporality of becoming: Care as an activity to support the being and becoming of the other. *Mind, Culture, and Activity, 0*(0), 1–21. https://doi.org/10.1080/10749039.2020.1745846

Raia, F., & Deng, M. (2015a). Is relational medicine the key to providing truly personalized high-tech modern medicine? *Personalized Medicine, 12*(1), 5–7.

Raia, F., & Deng, M. (2015b). *Relational medicine: Personalizing modern healthcare: The practice of high-tech medicine as a RelationalAct.* Imperial College Press World Scientific.

Raia, F., & Deng, M. C. (2016a). Mindfulness or recursive oscillatory processes of attunement? In *Mindfulness and Educating Citizens for Everyday Life* (pp. 235–257). SensePublishers, Rotterdam. https://doi.org/10.1007/978-94-6300-570-8_14

Raia, F., & Deng, M. C. (2016b). Artificial heart pumps: Bridging the gap between science, technology and personalized medicine by relational medicine. *Future Cardiology, 13*(1), 23–32. https://doi.org/10.2217/fca-2016-0020

Raia, F., Goodwin, M. H., & Deng, M. C. (2020). Forms of touch during medical encounters with an advanced heart failure (ADHF) doctor who practices relational medicine. *Social Interaction. Video-Based Studies of Human Sociality, 3*(1). https://doi.org/10.7146/si.v3i1.120259

Raia, F., Legados, L., Silacheva, I., Plotkin, J. B., Krishnan, S., & Deng, M. C. (2021). What is that's going on here? A multidimensional time concept is foundational to framing for decision making in situations of uncertainty. *Cultural Studies of Science Education, 16*, 881–913. https://doi.org/10.1007/s11422-021-10063-7

Raia, F., & Smith, M. S. (2020). Practitioners' noticing and know-how in multi-activity practice of patient care and teaching and learning. *Cognition and Instruction, 0*(0), 1–29. https://doi.org/10.1080/07370008.2020.1782411

Rao, P., Khalpey, Z., Smith, R., Burkhoff, D., & Kociol, R. D. (2018). Venoarterial extracorporeal membrane oxygenation for cardiogenic shock and cardiac arrest. *Circulation: Heart Failure, 11*(9), e004905. https://doi.org/10.1161/CIRCHEARTFAILURE.118. 004905

Richards, J., Elby, A., Luna, M. J., Robertson, A. D., Levin, D. M., & Nyeggen, C. G. (2020). Reframing the responsiveness challenge: A framing-anchored explanatory framework to account for irregularity in novice teachers' attention and responsiveness to student thinking. *Cognition and Instruction, 38*(2), 116–152. https://doi.org/10. 1080/07370008.2020.1729156

Ritchart, A., & Arvaniti, A. (2014). *The form and use of uptalk in Southern Californian English*. https://doi.org/10.21437/SPEECHPROSODY.2014-53

Robertson, M., Moir, J., Skelton, J., Dowell, J., & Cowan, S. (2011). When the business of sharing treatment decisions is not the same as shared decision making: A discourse analysis of decision sharing in general practice. *Health, 15*(1), 78–95. https://doi.org/ 10.1177/1363459309360788

Robertson, A. D., Richards, J., Elby, A., & Walkoe, J. (2016). Documenting variability within teacher attention and responsiveness to the substance of student thinking. In A. D. Robertson, R. Scherr, & D. Hammer (Eds.), Responsive Teaching in Science and Mathematics (pp. 227–247). New York, NY: Routledge.

Rocco, D., Pastore, M., Gennaro, A., Salvatore, S., Cozzolino, M., & Scorza, M. (2018). Beyond verbal behavior: An empirical analysis of speech rates in psychotherapy sessions. *Frontiers in Psychology, 9*. https://doi.org/10.3389/fpsyg.2018.00978

Ross, H., Abbey, S., Luca, E. D., Mauthner, O., McKeever, P., Shildrick, M., & Poole, J. (2010). What they say versus what we see: "Hidden" distress and impaired quality of life in heart transplant recipients. *The Journal of Heart and Lung Transplantation, 29*(10), 1142–1149. https://doi.org/10.1016/j.healun.2010.05.009

Rotenstein, L. S., Huckman, R. S., & Wagle, N. W. (2017). Making patients and doctors happier — The potential of patient-reported outcomes. *New England Journal of Medicine, 377*(14), 1309–1312. https://doi.org/10.1056/NEJMp1707537

Russ, R. S., & Luna, M. J. (2013). Inferring teacher epistemological framing from local patterns in teacher noticing. *Journal of Research in Science Teaching, 50*(3), 284–314. https://doi.org/10.1002/tea.21063

Sacks, H., Schegloff, E. A., & Jefferson, G. (1974). A simplest systematics for the organization of turn-taking for conversation. *Language, 50*(4), 696–735. https://doi.org/10.2307/412243

Sadala, M. L. A., Stolf, N. G., Bocchi, E. A., & Bicudo, M. A. V. (2013). Caring for heart transplant recipients: The lived experience of primary caregivers. *Heart & Lung, 42*(2), 120–125. https://doi.org/10.1016/j.hrtlng.2012.09.006

Salimbangon, A., Vucicevic, D., Lum, C., Chang, A., Khuu, T., Moore, M., Chand, R., Cadeiras, M., Kwon, M., Deng, M., Kamath, M., & DePasquale, E. (2019). Is there a mortality "weekend effect" in cardiac transplantation — a single center experience? *The Journal of Heart and Lung Transplantation, 38*(Suppl. 4), S397. https://doi.org/ 10.1016/j.healun.2019.01.1011

Schatzki, T. R., Knorr Cetina, K., & von Savigny, E. (2005). *The practice turn in contemporary theory*. Routledge.

Schegloff, E. A. (1987). Analyzing single episodes of interaction: An exercise in conversation analysis. *Social Psychology Quarterly, 50*(2), 101–114. JSTOR. https://doi.org/10.2307/2786745

Scott, R. L., Ratliff, N. B., Starling, R. C., & Young, J. B. (2001). Recurrence of giant cell myocarditis in cardiac allograft. *The Journal of Heart and Lung Transplantation, 20*(3), 375–380. https://doi.org/10.1016/S1053-2498(00)00314-4

Seem, D. L., Lee, I., Umscheid, C. A., Kuehnert, M. J., & United States Public Health Service. (2013). PHS guideline for reducing human immunodeficiency virus, hepatitis B virus, and hepatitis C virus transmission through organ transplantation. *Public Health Reports (Washington, D.C.: 1974), 128*(4), 247–343. https://doi.org/10.1177/003335491312800403

Sharp, L. A. (1995). Organ transplantation as a transformative experience: Anthropological insights into the restructuring of the self. *Medical Anthropology Quarterly, 9*(3), 357–389. https://doi.org/10.1525/maq.1995.9.3.02a00050

Sharp, L. A. (2006). *Strange harvest: Organ transplants, denatured bodies, and the transformed self*. University of California Press.

Sherin, M. G., & van Es, E. A. (2009). Effects of video club participation on teachers' professional vision. *Journal of Teacher Education, 60*(1), 20–37. https://doi.org/10.1177/0022487108328155

Shetty, P. A., Magazine, R., & Chogtu, B. (2021). Patient outlook on bedside teaching in a medical school. *Journal of Taibah University Medical Sciences, 16*(1), 50–56. https://doi.org/10.1016/j.jtumed.2020.10.002

Shildrick, M. (2011). *Imagining the heart: Incorporations, intrusions and identity*. https://doi.org/10.3366/SOMA.2012.0059

Shildrick, M. (2012). Hospitality and 'the gift of life': Reconfiguring the other in heart transplantation. In S. Gonzalez-Amal, G. Jagger, & K. Lennon (Eds.), *Embodied selves* (pp. 196–208). Palgrave Macmillan.

Shildrick, M. (2015). Staying alive: Affect, identity and anxiety in organ transplantation. *Body & Society, 21*(3), 20–41. https://doi.org/10.1177/1357034X15585886

Shildrick, M., McKeever, P., Abbey, S., Poole, J., & Ross, H. (2009). Troubling dimensions of heart transplantation. *Medical Humanities, 35*(1), 35–38. https://doi.org/10.1136/jmh.2008.001073

Silverman, D. (1997). *HIV counselling as social interaction*. Sage.

Silverman, D., & Peräkylä, A. (1990). AIDS counselling: The interactional organisation of talk about 'delicate' issues. *Sociology of Health & Illness, 12*(3), 293–318. https://doi.org/10.1111/1467-9566.ep11347251

Simpkin, A. L., & Schwartzstein, R. M. (2016). Tolerating uncertainty — The next medical revolution? *New England Journal of Medicine, 375*(18), 1713–1715. https://doi.org/10.1056/NEJMp1606402

Skelton, J. R., Wearn, A. M., & Hobbs, F. D. R. (2002). "I" and "we": A concordancing analysis of how doctors and patients use first person pronouns in primary care consultations. *Family Practice, 19*(5), 484–488. https://doi.org/10.1093/fampra/19.5.484

Speice, J., Harkness, J., Laneri, H., Frankel, R., Roter, D., Kornblith, A. B., Ahles, T., Winer, E., Fleishman, S., Luber, P., Zevon, M., Mcquellon, R., Trief, P., Finkel, J.,

Spira, J., Greenberg, D., Rowland, J., & Holland, J. C. (2000). Involving family members in cancer care: Focus group considerations of patients and oncological providers. *Psycho-Oncology, 9*(2), 101–112. https://doi.org/10.1002/(SICI)1099-1611(200003/04)9:2$<$101::AID-PON435$>$3.0.CO;2-D

Sterponi, L., Zucchermaglio, C., Fatigante, M., & Alby, F. (2019). Structuring times and activities in the oncology visit. *Social Science & Medicine, 228*, 211–222. https://doi.org/10.1016/j.socscimed.2019.03.036

Stevens, R., & Hall, R. (1998). Disciplined perception: Learning to see in technoscience. In M. Lampert & M. L. Blunk (Eds.), *Talking mathematics in school: Studies of teaching and learning* (pp. 107–149). Cambridge University Press.

Stivers, T., & Heritage, J. (2001). Breaking the sequential mold: Answering 'more than the question' during comprehensive history taking. *Text–Interdisciplinary Journal for the Study of Discourse, 21*(1–2). https://doi.org/10.1515/text.1.21.1-2.151

Strang, S., Henoch, I., Danielson, E., Browall, M., & Melin-Johansson, C. (2014). Communication about existential issues with patients close to death — Nurses' reflections on content, process and meaning. *Psycho-Oncology, 23*(5), 562–568. https://doi.org/10.1002/pon.3456

Streeck, J. (2017). *Self-making man: A day of action, life, and language.* Cambridge University Press.

Streeck, J., & Mehus, S. (2005). Microethnography: The study of practices. In K. L. Fitch & R. E. Sanders (Eds.), *Handbook of language and social interaction* (pp. 381–404). Lawrence Erlbaum Associates Publishers.

Strout, T. D., Hillen, M., Gutheil, C., Anderson, E., Hutchinson, R., Ward, H., Kay, H., Mills, G. J., & Han, P. K. J. (2018). Tolerance of uncertainty: A systematic review of health and healthcare-related outcomes. *Patient Education and Counseling, 101*(9), 1518–1537. https://doi.org/10.1016/j.pec.2018.03.030

Suchman, A. L., Markakis, K., Beckman, H. B., & Frankel, R. (1997). A model of empathic communication in the medical interview. *JAMA, 277*(8), 678–682. https://doi.org/10.1001/jama.1997.03540320082047

Supelana, C., Annunziato, R. A., Kaplan, D., Helcer, J., Stuber, M. L., & Shemesh, E. (2016). PTSD in solid organ transplant recipients: Current understanding and future implications. *Pediatric Transplantation, 20*(1), 23–33. https://doi.org/10.1111/petr.12628

Swilder, A. (2005). What anchors cultural practices. In T. R. Schatzki, K. Knorr Cetina, & E. von Savigny (Eds.), *The practice turn in contemporary theory.* Routledge.

Tannen, D. (1993). *Framing in discourse.* Oxford University Press.

Tannen, D., & Wallat, C. (1987). Interactive frames and knowledge schemas in interaction: Examples from a medical examination/interview. *Social Psychology Quarterly, 50*(2), 205. https://doi.org/10.2307/2786752

Ten Have, P. (1991). Talk and institution: A reconsideration of the 'asymmetry' of doctor patient interaction. In *Talk and Social Structure: Studies in Ethnomethodology and Conversation Analysis* (pp. 138–163).

Throop, C. J. (2003). Articulating experience. *Anthropological Theory, 3*(2), 219–241. https://doi.org/10.1177/1463499603003002006

Throop, C. J., & Zahavi, D. (2020). Dark and bright empathy: Phenomenological and anthropological reflections. *Current Anthropology, 61*(3), 283–303. https://doi.org/10.1086/708844

Timmermans, S., & Almeling, R. (2009). Objectification, standardization, and commodification in health care: A conceptual readjustment. *Social Science & Medicine, 69*(1), 21–27. https://doi.org/10.1016/j.socscimed.2009.04.020
Timmermans, S., & Angell, A. (2001). Evidence-based medicine, clinical uncertainty, and learning to doctor. *Journal of Health and Social Behavior, 42*(4), 342–359. https://doi.org/10.2307/3090183
Timmermans, S., & Mauck, A. (2005). The promises and pitfalls of evidence-based medicine. *Health Affairs, 24*(1), 18–28. https://doi.org/10.1377/hlthaff.24.1.18
Timmermans, S., Tietbohl, C., & Skaperdas, E. (2017). Narrating uncertainty: Variants of uncertain significance (VUS) in clinical exome sequencing. *BioSocieties, 12*(3), 439–458. https://doi.org/10.1057/s41292-016-0020-5
Tonelli, M. R., & Upshur, R. E. G. (2019). A philosophical approach to addressing uncertainty in medical education. *Academic Medicine, 94*(4), 507–511. https://doi.org/10.1097/ACM.0000000000002512
Torres, C. A. (2008). *Education and neoliberal globalization.* Routledge.
United Network for Organ Sharing. (2021). *New OPTN policies to align with updated U.S. Public Health Service Guideline.* Author. https://unos.org/news/policy-changes/new-optn-policies-to-align-with-updated-u-s-public-health-service-guideline/
van Nijnatten, C., & Suoninen, E. (2013). Delicacy. In C. Hall, K. Juhila, M. Matarese, & C. Van Nijnatten (Eds.), *Analysing social work communication: Discourse in practice* (pp. 136–153). Routledge.
Volk, M. L., Wilk, A. R., Wolfe, C., & Kaul, D. R. (2017). The "PHS increased risk" Label is associated with nonutilization of hundreds of organs per year. *Transplantation, 101*(7), 1666–1669. https://doi.org/10.1097/TP.0000000000001673
Voltolini, A., Salvato, G., Frigerio, M., Cipriani, M., Perna, E., Pisu, M., & Mazza, U. (2020). Psychological outcomes of left ventricular assist device long-term treatment: A 2-year follow-up study. *Artificial Organs, 44*(1), 67–71. https://doi.org/10.1111/aor.13531
Vucicevic, D., Honoris, L., Raia, F., & Deng, M. (2018). Current indications for transplantation: Stratification of severe heart failure and shared decision-making. *Annals of Cardiothoracic Surgery, 7*(1), 56–66. https://doi.org/10.21037/acs.2017.12.01
Warren, P. (2016). *Uptalk: The phenomenon of rising intonation.* Cambridge University Press.
Wayne, S., Dellmore, D., Serna, L., Jerabek, R., Timm, C., & Kalishman, S. (2011). The association between intolerance of ambiguity and decline in medical students' attitudes toward the underserved. *Academic Medicine: Journal of the Association of American Medical Colleges, 86*(7), 877–882. https://doi.org/10.1097/ACM.0b013e31821dac01
Webb, H. (2010). *The Medieval Heart.* Yale University Press.
Weber, M. (1978). *Economy and Society: An Outline of Interpretive Sociology.* Univ of California Press.
Weijts, W., Houtkoop, H., & Mullen, P. (1993). Talking delicacy: Speaking about sexuality during gynaecological consultations. *Sociology of Health & Illness, 15*(3), 295–314. https://doi.org/10.1111/1467-9566.ep10490531
Wellbery, C. (2010). The value of medical uncertainty? *The Lancet, 375*(9727), 1686–1687. https://doi.org/10.1016/S0140-6736(10)60725-8

West, A. F., & West, R. R. (2002). Clinical decision-making: Coping with uncertainty. *Postgraduate Medical Journal, 78*(920), 319–321. https://doi.org/10.1136/pmj.78.920.319

West, C. (1984). Medical misfires: Mishearings, misgivings, and misunderstandings in physician-patient dialogues. *Discourse Processes, 7*(2), 107–134. https://doi.org/10.1080/01638538409544586

Whitney, S. N., McGuire, A. L., & McCullough, L. B. (2004). A typology of shared decision making, informed consent, and simple consent. *Annals of Internal Medicine, 140*(1), 54. https://doi.org/10.7326/0003-4819-140-1-200401060-00012

Wirtz, V., Cribb, A., & Barber, N. (2006). Patient–doctor decision-making about treatment within the consultation — A critical analysis of models. *Social Science & Medicine, 62*(1), 116–124. https://doi.org/10.1016/j.socscimed.2005.05.017

Worrall, J. (2007). Evidence in medicine and evidence-based medicine. *Philosophy Compass, 2*(6), 981–1022. https://doi.org/10.1111/j.1747-9991.2007.00106.x

Wrathall, M. (2000). Background practices, capacities, and Heideggerian disclosure. In *Heidegger, Coping, and Cognitive Science: Essays in Honor of Hubert L. Dreyfus* (Vol. 2, pp. 93–114).

Wray, C. M., & Loo, L. K. (2015). The diagnosis, prognosis, and treatment of medical uncertainty. *Journal of Graduate Medical Education, 7*(4), 523–527. https://doi.org/10.4300/JGME-D-14-00638.1

You, J. J., Aleksova, N., Ducharme, A., MacIver, J., Mielniczuk, L., Fowler, R. A., Demers, C., Clarke, B., Parent, M.-C., Toma, M., Strachan, P. H., Farand, P., Isaac, D., Zieroth, S., Swinton, M., Jiang, X., Day, A. G., Heyland, D. K., & Ross, H. J. (2017). Barriers to goals of care discussions with patients who have advanced heart failure: results of a multicenter survey of hospital-based cardiology clinicians. *Journal of Cardiac Failure, 23*(11), 786–793. https://doi.org/10.1016/j.cardfail.2017.06.003

Zikmund-Fisher, B. J. (2013). The right tool is what they need, not what we have: A taxonomy of appropriate levels of precision in patient risk communication. *Medical Care Research and Review, 70*(Suppl. 1), 37S–49S. https://doi.org/10.1177/1077558712458541

Zulman, D. M., Haverfield, M. C., Shaw, J. G., Brown-Johnson, C. G., Schwartz, R., Tierney, A. A., Zionts, D. L., Safaeinili, N., Fischer, M., Thadaney Israni, S., Asch, S. M., & Verghese, A. (2020). Practices to foster physician presence and connection with patients in the clinical encounter. *JAMA, 323*(1), 70–81. https://doi.org/10.1001/jama.2019.19003

INDEX

Note: **Bold** page numbers refer to tables; *Italic* page numbers refer to figures and page numbers followed by "n" denote footnotes.

Return of Spontaneous Circulation
(ROSC), 122
revascularization, 47
rheumatology team, 83
rhizomatic approach, 63
rhythmic cardio-compression, 122
Right Ventricular Assist Device (RVAD),
59, 116, 151
rising intonation, 70
role distributions, 102, 158, 179
ROSC. *see* Return of Spontaneous
Circulation (ROSC)
RVAD. *see* Right Ventricular Assist
Device (RVAD)

S

safe spaces, 176
scenario planning, 110
science experiment, 81
scientific evidence, 48
Selection Committee, 109, 133, 173
self-repairs, 78
semantic distinction, 180
sense of urgency, 92
shared decision-making process, 2
shared disappointment, 96
shared frameworks, 182
silences, 56, 100
single-case analysis, 36
"sinking in," 178
S/IT. *see* surgical/interventional therapy
(S/IT)
skill levels, 174
social interaction, 134
social life, 134
social organization, 134
social positioning, 66
Society for Medical Decision Making, 1
soft power, 76, 179
speech pattern, 142
speech rate, 70, 142
spiritual connections, 162
spiritual life, 171
stakeholders, 10
stating, 138
stent implantation, 47

students, 8, 21
surgeon-patient relationship, 116
surgeons, 118
    cogen session, 129
    instability, 123
    next generation, 129
    urgency, 123
surgical/interventional therapy (S/IT), 48
surgical perspective, 119
survival rates, *41*
SVR. *see* Systemic Vascular Resistance
(SVR)
Swan Ganz catheter, 79
synchronization with the Other, 171
Systemic Vascular Resistance (SVR), 104

T

tacrolimus, 86, 134
TAH. *see* Total Artificial Heart (TAH)
talking down, 72
talk-in-interaction method, 31
Tannen, Deborah, 17
taxonomy, uncertainty, 60n8
teaching hospital, 127, 129
team, 2
technicity paradigm, 14, 15
telemedicine practices, 18
temporal horizon, 142
textbook answer, 124
theatrical performance, 134
therapeutic plan, 86
time-dependent frame, 147
timeline, 140
timing, heart transplant, 109
Total Artificial Heart (TAH), 65, 116
trainees, 66
transcripts symbols, 35
transformation, 130
transitive verb, 138
transplantation, 101–104
transplantation listing process, 99
transplant list, 39
transplant Olympics, 85
tree-like taxonomy, 60
trustful relations, 170, 173
trusting relationship, 176

U

ultrasound examination, 122
uncertainty, 2, 22–27, 37, 54, 60, 63,
  177–178
    ambiguity, 25
    complexity, 25
    domains of, 177
    in-training physicians' struggle, 22
    issues of, 26–27
    layers of, 74
    locus of, 27
    in medical decision-making, 23
    medical school training, 22
    probability, 25
    of source, 25–26
    taxonomy, 26, 60n8
    theoretical concept, 22
    tolerance and physicians, 23–24
United Network for Organ Sharing
  (UNOS), 88, 115
UNOS. see United Network for Organ
  Sharing (UNOS)
UNOS 1A list, 79
UNOS requirements, 62
UNOS Status 7, 115
unratified hearers, 67
uptalk, 70
urgent, 105, 131

V

VAD. see VentricularAssistDevice (VAD)
VA-ECMO. see Venoarterial
  Extracorporeal Membrane Oxygenator
  (VA-ECMO)

values-based preferences, 48
value system, 172
vascular resistance, 97
Venoarterial Extracorporeal Membrane
  Oxygenator (VA-ECMO), 6, 157, 167
venous cannula, 122
Ventricular Assist Devices (VADs), 1, 115
ventricular fibrillation, 37, 38
ventricular tachyarrhythmia, 37, 38
ventricular tachycardia (V-tach), 40, 148
ventricular tachycardia ablation, 47
video- and audio recordings, 30
Virgil, 83
viruses, 58
Volkswagens, 172
V-tach. see ventricular tachycardia
  (V-tach)
v-tach/v-fib, 7

W

way of life, 78
weekend effect, 126–131, 127
Wellbery, Caroline Dr., 22
white coats, 90
world of medicine, 127

Z

zapped energy, 91

www.ingramcontent.com/pod-product-compliance
Lightning Source LLC
Chambersburg PA
CBHW050559190326
41458CB00007B/2106

* 9 7 8 9 8 1 1 2 5 4 6 7 3 *